September 11

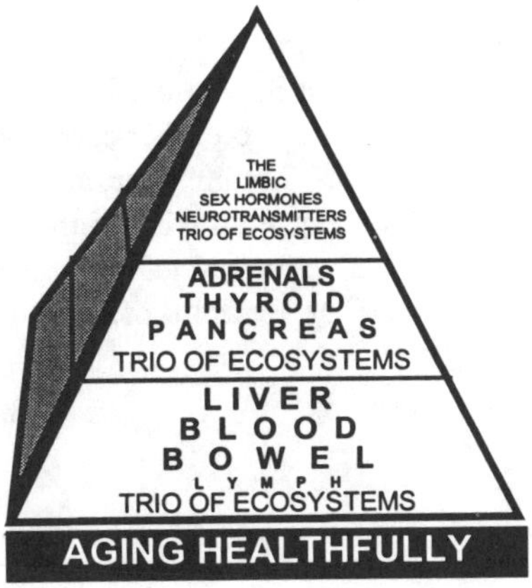

September Eleven, 2005
© Majid Ali, 2002
All Rights Reserved

No part of this work may be reproduced or transmitted in any form or by any means, electronic or mechanical, including photocopy, recording, taping, or any information storage and retrieval mechanism presently known or to be invented, without permission in writing from the publisher, except by a reviewer who wishes to quote excerpts from this volume in reference to a review written for publication in a magazine, newspaper or broadcast.

Treatments and guidelines written of in this book are not to be performed as a self-help guideline. Any change in your medical regiment should be discussed with your physician.

Library of Congress Catalog Card Number
On File

ISBN 1-879131-22-6

Ali, Majid
September 11, 2005
Majid Ali.—1st ed.

Includes bibliographical references and index
1. The September Eleven syndrome
2. The September canaries
3. The human canaries
4. Oxygen dysfunction
5. Dysfunctional oxygen metabolism
6. The Pyramid of Human Ecosystems

10 9 8 7 6 5 4 3 2 1

Aging Healthfully, Inc.
140 West End Avenue Suite 1H
New York, NY 10023
1-800-633-6226

SEPTEMBER ELEVEN, 2005

In September 2005, there were over 250,000 human canaries in the City. They had initially endured the terror and toxicity of collapsed Twin Towers, then developed immune dysfunctions, and eventually collapsed into the Malady. They suffered in silence, shunned by their doctors, neglected by the City officials, and considered malingerers by their families and friends.

Majid Ali, M.D.

Dedicated to all the human canaries of this world who suffer in silence and whose physical afflictions are ignored by their doctors simply because the symptom-complexes do not fit into textbook classifications of diseases.

There are no controversies in medicine, only levels of understanding and enlightenment

September 11, 2005

by

Majid Ali, M.D.

President and Professor of Medicine,
Capital University of Integrative Medicine,
Washington, D.C.

Former Associate Professor of Pathology (adj.),
College of Physicians and Surgeons,
Columbia University, New York, NY

Editor, The Journal of Integrative Medicine

Former, President of Medical Staff and Chief Pathologist, Holy Name Hospital, Teaneck, New Jersey

President, The Institute of Integrative Medicine,
New York and Denville, New Jersey

Fellow, Royal College of Physicians & Surgeons
of England

Diplomate, American Boards of Anatomic
and Clinical Pathology

Diplomate, American Board of Environmental
Medicine

Aging Healthfully, Inc.
www.aginghealthfully.com

This book is organized in five parts:

In September 2001, over four million people in the City suffered from anxiety and sleep problems. The doctors freely dispensed anxiety and sleeping pills. The City officials also rose to the occasion and arranged for free counseling.

In September 2002, over 500,000 people in the City suffered from recurrent infections, digestive disorders, undue tiredness, and mood problems. The doctors worked feverishly to uncover the underlying cause and develop effective therapies for the epidemic.

In September 2003, over 250,000 people in the City suffered from disabling fatigue, unrelenting muscle pain, and brain fog. The doctors were tired of listening to a plethora of complaints which they neither understood nor could treat. The City officials had also lost interest. Their families and friends were baffled.

In September 2005, there were over 250,000 human canaries in the City and an untold number in the country. They had initially endured the terror and toxicity of collapsed Twin Towers, then developed immune dysfunctions, and eventually collapsed into the Malady. They suffered in silence, shunned by their doctors, neglected by the City officials, and considered malingerers by their families and friends.

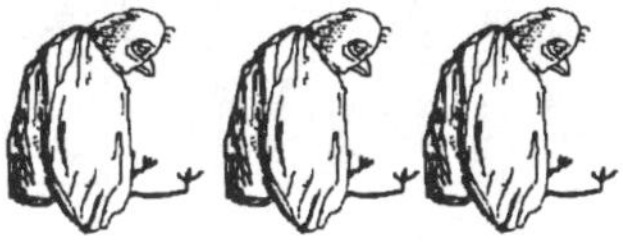

In September 2005, there were also over 115,000 Gulf War canaries in the country. They also suffered in silence, shunned by their doctors, neglected by the Department of Defense, and considered malingerers by their families and friends.

The birds of passage
Arrive with a broken
Wing,

Though
Are lifted by God
So high and
"Low"

To experience the heart
Of everything.

The mind surely becomes disarrayed
When the Teacher is out
Of sight.

Hafiz
(Sufi Shams-ud-din Mohammad Hafiz 1320-1389.
From a translation by Daniel Landkinsky.)

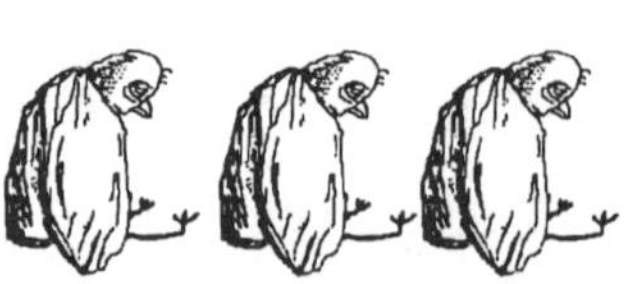

Acknowledgment

I am profoundly grateful to the medical, nursing, and administrative staffs of the Institute of Integrative Medicine who for years have worked hard to create an environment in which I see patients and conduct my research. I am also indebted to Barry Weiner, Jerald Finnie, M.D., Dolores Finnie, and Amy Lang for their kind assistance in reviewing the manuscript.

Part 1

How the epidemic of September Eleven Syndrome began

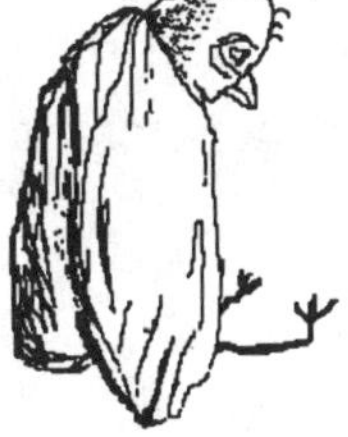

Two Flashes, Two Epidemics

As the first of the two Twin Towers began to collapse, I saw in a flash that it was the beginning of a very long story—the same story I had seen in a flash ten years earlier in the first images of terror and toxicity of burning oil fields in the Gulf War.

In 2001, ten years after the Gulf War, there were over 115,000 victims of the Gulf War syndrome in the country. They lived severely diminished lives, shunned by doctors, neglected by the Department of Defense, and considered malingerers by their families and friends.

In 2005, four years after the collapse of the Twin Towers, there were over 250,000 victims of the September Eleven syndrome in the City. They also lived severely diminished lives, shunned by doctors, neglected by the City officials, and considered malingerers by their families and friends.

In 1991, nearly 700,000 men and women were involved in the Persian Gulf conflict. Later, more than one of every ten such persons developed the Gulf War syndrome.

In 2001, over two and one-half millions people in metropolitan New York were exposed to the unrelenting terror and toxicity of the Twin Towers inferno. Later, more than one of every ten such persons developed the September Eleven syndrome.

The Human Canaries

In old mining days, miners carried canaries in cages deep into their mine shafts. The birds were a sort of intelligence system. If there were poisonous gases in the shafts, the birds would warn the miners. When the birds collapsed or died, the miners knew there were toxic gases in the shaft even though they could not smell them. They left the birds and ran out to escape the poisonous mine gases.

I consider persons with the Gulf War and September Eleven syndromes to be human canaries. They are more vulnerable to environmental toxins than others. They are more sensitive to functional nutritional deficiencies than others. Their cells and tissues are more readily injured by oxidative stress then others. They develop the oxygen disorder sooner than others. The oxygen disorder then leads to weakness of the immune system, chronic ill, health, fatigue, and problems of mood, memory, and mentation.

The anguish and suffering of the Gulf War and September Eleven canaries cannot be understood until their constitutional weakness is recognized. Nor can they be treated properly until their special needs for nutritional support and detoxification are addressed.

The Oxygen Disorder

The term oxygen disorder appears throughout this book. Below, I explain the basic oxygen disorder of the September canaries with a simple analogy.

A car engine mixes fuel and oxygen to produce energy. A properly maintained engine performs without generating excessive toxic exhaust. An engine clogged with soot produces less energy and more toxic fumes. The basic difference between the two is that fuel is completely burned in the first instance, leaving no toxic residue behind, whereas in the second car incomplete combustion leads to generation of excess toxic residue.

Like the good engine, a healthy person uses oxygen to extract clean energy from his meal. By contrast, a human canary with an oxygen disorder cannot do so without producing excess toxic waste which, in turn, causes fatigue and immune weakness.

The presence of the oxygen disorder can be easily established by doing urine analysis for toxic acids.

The Terror and Toxicity of the Gulf War

Back in 1991, in the first TV pictures of the Gulf War conflagration, I recognized the dangerous combination of toxicity and terror. I realized then that the soldiers with hidden weaknesses of the immune system—the human canaries, in my language—would develop chronic and clinically debilitating immune dysfunction. I knew well how those sick persons would become the Gulf War canaries.

In those pictures, I also saw how the story of the veterans would unfold. Initially, the military doctors would treat them vigorously with deep concern, diligence, and empathy. Congress would be loud in its support for them as well. The military would soon call in civil medical experts to assist and guide them in uncovering the nature of the illness. They would not bother to seek advice from nutritionists and environmental doctors. Within months, medical journals would dub the problem as the Gulf War syndrome and attribute it to stress of the war. Antianxiety pills and antidepressants would be liberally prescribed. The drugs would be of little help. More journal reports would follow claiming that there is no evidence of chemical or immune injury in the syndrome. Next, some people would pronounce that the syndrome is caused by some microbes and would administer potent—and toxic—antibiotics in large amounts. There would be limited benefits in some cases, but serious long-term consequences in most others.

The victims of the war epidemic would go on to develop many symptom-complexes that would confound medical experts. Their special needs of nutrition would be ignored. The stresses on their bowels, blood, and livers would go unrecognized. The immune injury and oxygen dysfunction inflicted by the war events would be dismissed as an imagined disorder of troubled minds. In months or years, the Gulf War syndrome would be seen as a combination of hypochondria, obsessive-compulsive disorder, and stress syndrome. Years later, there would be thousands of veterans living severely diminished lives, shunned by doctors, neglected by the Department of Defense, and considered malingerers by their families and friends.

The Terror and Toxicity of the Twin Towers

In 2001, in the first pictures of the collapsing Twin Towers, I again saw how the terror and toxicity of the inferno would cause chronic and debilitating immune injury and oxygen dysfunctions. I realized then that hundreds of thousands of persons with weak immune systems would be turned into the September canaries. I also saw how their stories would unfold.

Hundreds of tons of PCBs and related toxic chemicals were used in the manufacture of electrical wires and other equipment installed in the Towers complex. There were enormous quantities of Freon and other chemicals in air conditioner units in the complex. What other classes of toxic materials were present in the buildings at that time was anybody's guess. I knew that most of those chemicals would be incompletely burned and many converted into yet more toxic substances—Freon turning into nerve gas was just one such horrifying possibility. Dioxin—one of the most potent carcinogens known—and other highly poisonous benzene derivatives were detected. The winds spread the toxic chemicals over large areas, but the poisons did not escape into outer space. It was a case of what goes up comes down. Winds only dispersed the toxins and widened the contaminated toxic zone. NASA flew missions with remote-sensing aircraft over Ground Zero. Onboard instruments detected a large number of synthetic chemicals and metals. Computer-generated maps of the area pinpointed dozens of hot spots, reaching up to 1,300 degrees Fahrenheit.

I recognized how dangerous such massive chemical exposures would be when added to the chemistry of overwhelming fear—not only of what had been witnessed, but also of the unknown that might follow.

In that flash, I also clearly saw how the story of the victims of the terror and toxicity of the Twin Towers would unfold. Initially, the City doctors would treat them with deep concern, diligence, and empathy. The City officials will be loud in their support for them as well. Then they will call upon experts in stress management from other cities. They will not bother to seek advice from nutritionists and environmental doctors. Within months, medical journals will dub the problem as the September Eleven syndrome and attribute it to stress of the Twin Tower havoc. Antianxiety pills and antidepressants will be liberally prescribed. The drugs will help but little. More journal reports will follow claiming that there is no evidence of chemical or immune injury in the syndrome. Next, some people will pronounce that the syndrome is caused by some microbes and administer potent—and toxic—antibiotics in large amounts. There would be limited benefits in some cases but serious long-term consequences in most others.

The September canaries would go on to develop many symptom-complexes that will confound medical experts. Their special needs of nutrition would be ignored. The stresses on their bowels, blood, and livers will go unrecognized. The immune injury and oxygen dysfunctions inflicted by the Twin Tower catastrophe would be dismissed as imagined troubles of troubled minds. In months or years, it would be pronounced by the leading medical journals that the September Eleven syndrome is nothing more than varying combinations of hypochondria, obsessive-compulsive disorder, and stress syndrome. Years later, there would be thousands of victims of the syndrome living severely diminished lives, shunned by doctors, neglected by the City officials, and considered malingerers by their families and friends.

The Gulf War Syndrome Was Predictable

And it was predicted. Its existence was denied by some for pseudoscientific reasons. Others neglected the Gulf War canaries for selfish financial and/or political ends.

The September Eleven Syndrome Was Predictable

And it was predicted. Its existence was denied by some for pseudoscientific reasons. Others neglected the September canaries for selfish financial and/or political ends.

Gulf War Syndrome—Who's Addressing the Issue?

The characteristics of the Gulf War syndrome were entirely predictable. And those were predicted. Consider the following text from the September 13, 1995, issue of *Navy News*:

> Long before the first veterans returned from the Persian Gulf Dr. Majid Ali, associate professor of pathology at the College of Physicians and Surgeons at Columbia University in New York, and Director of the Department of Pathology, Immunology and Laboratories at Holy Name Hospital in Teaneck, NJ, predicted five outcomes.
>
> * That a large number of service men and women in the Persian Gulf region would return with a variety of chronic environmental, immune and stress related problems;

* The disabling fatigue would be a dominant clinical feature while other symptoms would include recurrent infection; food allergy reactions, abdominal problems, disorders of mood and memory, and skin rashes, among others;
* That sick veterans would initially be dismissed as malingerers and labeled with various psychiatric diagnoses and prescribed large doses of mind numbing drugs;
* That the chronic health disorders of these veterans would worsen with multiple drug therapies; and
* That when everything else failed, these veterans would be prescribed long term broad spectrum antibiotic therapy that would play further havoc with their bowel systems.

Five years later these predictions are now observable fact. Headlines debate the cause and fate of those men and women who left healthy and returned home sick—nearly 75,000 at last count.

Not surprisingly, the voice of *Navy News* was drowned in the noise made by *Nature* and *The New England Journal of Medicine.*

The Victims of a Pernicious Idea

The Gulf War canaries were victims of a pernicious idea of the prevailing medicine—that every form of ill health has to conform to a textbook description of a disease. There had never been a war before in which the soldiers were so massively exposed to toxic chemicals, were terrorized by the high probability of biologic warfare, and faced predictions of nearly 100,000 casualties. The one-bug/one-disease/one-drug model of medical thinking was utterly irrelevant to those caught in the Persian Gulf conflict. And yet, when many veterans of that war returned sick, the military doctors and their civilian consultants looked for one disease caused by one chemical or one bug. Unable to reach a consensus on a single disease, they told everyone that there was really nothing wrong with the ill Gulf War veterans. That pernicious idea wrought havoc on the sick veterans. The doctors everywhere concluded that the Gulf War syndrome was an imagined malady of troubled minds. The victims were simply ignored. Consider the following quote from the October 9, 2000, issue of *Nature*:

> The problem with declaring that there is a Gulf War syndrome is that the research suggests that there is not.

An amazing display of naivete! And that from arguably the most prestigious science journal in the world. Whose research was it? Was it of experts who were looking for a *recognized disease* in the ill veterans but could not find any? Or was it of doctors who refused to examine the clear evidence of excessive oxidative injury to cells and body fluids and an oxygen disorder? The evidence of those disorders was certainly clear to me. Now consider another quote from the same issue of *Nature*:

> The US Congress should stop pushing researchers to invent a medical definition for Gulf War syndrome, the collection of maladies associated with veterans of the 1991 conflict in the Persian Gulf....although some of those exposures could be linked to acute symptoms, there was insufficient evidence to link any of them to chronic health problems.

Nature was distressed because the *collection of maladies* in veterans does not fit into a definition of an acceptable disease in the prevailing—and scientifically frivolous—one-disease/one-diagnosis/one-drug model of diseases. So it wanted Congress to stop people from pushing for answers. That poured more salt on the wounds of the sick.

The Gulf War syndrome, indeed, was a highly complex disorder. What dismayed me about *Nature's* position most was that it refused to accept that complexity and the challenge posed by it. By contrast, the journal had no difficulty accepting complexity in the extinction of many marine species caused by cumulative toxicity of environmental pollutants in coastal and ocean waters.

Now consider *The New England Journal of Medicine*. It took positions just as silly as those of *Nature*. An editorial published in its November 14, 1996, issue, included the following:

> Our troops received numerous immunizations and carried protective suits and pyridostigmine to use in case of exposure to nerve gas. They were exposed to heat, dust, insects, parasites, pesticides, fumes, fuels,

> and thick smoke. For weeks many lived with the dense residue from burning petroleum coating their skin.

So the *Journal* acknowledged an impressive, though partial, list of agents that could have caused chronic and debilitating problems of excessive oxidation and oxygen dysfunction. It underscored the length of periods of exposure, further emphasizing the problem. Next, its display of lack of common sense fully matched that of *Nature.* Consider the following quote from the same editorial:

> Physicians who care for these ailing veterans must resist the pressure to diagnose a disease for which scientific evidence is lacking.

Resist the pressure to diagnose a disease! The *Journal* did not encourage its readers to look deeper into the molecular basis of the suffering in veterans. Rather, it exhorted them not to diagnose any disease. Intellectual bankruptcy persisted. Like *Nature* before it, it engaged in the folly of denying the illness of veterans because it could not find a specific disease. It completely ignored the fundamental issues of cumulative terror and toxicity and how that dangerous combination leads to unrelenting oxidative injury and oxygen dysfunction, which then fan their own fires. The *Journal* was not willing to deal with the complexity of the sick veterans any more than *Nature*.

Next, *The New England Journal of Medicine* made an even more startling statement in that editorial. Consider the following quote:

> ....it may be impossible for science to ever establish whether serving in the Persian Gulf War really caused

a disease that produces only a wide range of symptoms.

May be impossible for science ever to establish! It fascinated me how the *Journal* reversed itself—seemingly without recognizing its turnabout—and conceded the possiblity of something being truly wrong with the sick veterans.

Who had the courage to challenge *Nature* and *The New England Journal of Medicine*? Congress, insurance companies, medical boards, and doctors were misled by medical journals —doctors, albeit not fully recognizing their role, contributed to the neglect of the sick veterans.

Then I thought that the sins of *Nature* may be overlooked. Those who write for it about matters of complexity in nature are true scientists without investment in the medical industrial complex. The *Journal* simply failed to recognize the fixation of its doctor-writers with the names of diseases. I could not show such generosity of the mind for *The New England Journal of Medicine*—its writers, I knew only too well, worshiped at the sacred altar of their one-bug/one-disease/one-drug god. They could not be drawn into the matters of poisoned cellular enzymes and of cells being choked by the oxygen disorder.

The Web, the Kaleidoscope, and the September Canaries

The characteristics of the September syndrome were also predictable. And those were predicted. Below, I reproduce some text from an article I wrote about the September canaries in December 2001:

> A full comprehension of three fundamental aspects of the human condition is required to clearly understand the health/dis-ease/disease continuum and the plight of the September canaries:
>
> 1. Human biology is an enormous web. Everything in that web is connected to everything else;
> 2. It is a panoramic kaleidoscope. When something in that kaleidoscope changes in one way, everything in it changes in some way; and
> 3. Both the web and the kaleidoscope are reflections of Nature's preoccupation with complementarity and contrariety.
>
> The September Eleven syndrome cannot be understood without understanding the above. And I am afraid it will not be.
>
> In the prevailing deterministic-reductionistic medicine in the City, all notions of disease causation and treatment are based on an assumption that all

atoms, molecules, and cells play *fixed and consistent* roles in health and disease. That assumption is without scientific merit. In reality, all elements in the human body take on changing roles under varying ecologic conditions. The worlds of genes, hormones, neurotransmitters, and mediator molecules of injury and healing responses are far too complex to be reduced to banalities, as is commonly done by the City doctors. The interactions between foreign synthetic chemicals and the body's own native substances cannot be understood—and clinically managed by the reductionistic one-bug/one-disease/one-drug model of diseases. That is the crux of the problem. The September Eleven syndrome can be neither understood nor prevented by the prevailing thinking among the doctors in the City.

I recognize that the practitioners of the prevailing one-chemical/one-disease/one-drug model of disease have no use for my broader—and clinically essential—concepts of Nature's preoccupation with structural and functional complementarity and contrariety. Taking the lead from the officials of the Environmental Protection Agency, the doctors dismiss the possibility that the *cumulative* chemical load of toxins from the Twin Towers caused the September Eleven syndrome. That was not unexpected for me. Nor am I surprised when the doctors vehemently rejected the idea that *cumulative* nutrient support administered by injections and intravenous infusions can facilitate detoxification and prevention of the syndrome.

But to prevent an enormous epidemic of a Gulf War-like syndrome, we physicians must understand and put to clinical use the twin themes of cellular multifunctionality and *functional relatedness* among human ecosystems. I am afraid that may turn out to be wishful thinking on my part.

When writing the above piece for our web site, I had little hope that my warning would be heeded. And it was not.

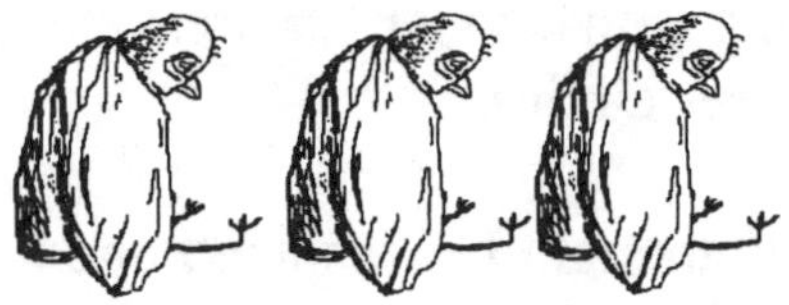

Spinning from one thread
that hung from the silk mandala,
I watched until they fell
As our bodies someday will,
Panting like a great falling star.

Hafiz

(Sofi Shams-ud-din Mohammad Hafiz 1320-1389. From a translation by Daniel Landkinsky.)

Not Impressed

The New England Journal of Medicine was not impressed by the woes of the September canaries—just as it had not been with the plight of the Gulf War canaries.

Two months after the havoc, in an editorial published in the November 15, 2001, issue, it included the following words:

> We are living with new threats to health, new worries, and new uncertainties.

New uncertainties! I thought I saw some hope for a change. Perhaps those *new* uncertainties will encourage the *Journal* to look beyond its subservience to the one-bug/one-disease/one-drug model—and, in that case, make an exception. Perhaps it would not dismiss the problems of the September canaries as an exaggerated stress response that turned into a psychiatric disorder. The *Journal* continued:

> In addressing these uncertainties, physicians' response should be rational and based on the knowledge and values that are fundamental to the mission of the health care professions.

Should be rational! Translation: One bug/one-disease/one-drug model of diagnosis and treatment. I realized I had been wrong about the *Journal* one more time. The *Journal* was concerned about the rationality of its readers—doctors, health officials, and insurance carriers—because it seemed to sense that it was going to witness a repeat of the Gulf War events. It seemed to suspect that many in the City will become irrational and claim that they were victims of the

September Eleven horrors. It was afraid that their irrationality could affect the rationality of its readers. Why else would it caution its readers to be rational if it did not think they would be taken advantage of by those who had lost their rationality?

It did not escape my notice that the *Journal* had cautioned not only doctors but all others in the health care professions. It was ever so mindful of its advertisement revenues. There were no drugs that could detoxify the liver. None to restore impaired oxygen metabolism.

In the years that followed, the *Journal* reiterated its position on many occasions. Those who claimed they were toxic, it asserted, were toxic only in their minds. Those who insisted their immune system had been injured by the events of September eleven, 2001, it warned, had lost their rationality. They merely suffered from the post-traumatic stress syndrome. What they really needed were compassion, psychotherapy and antidepressants.

The *Journal* showed no interest in exploring the possibility that the immune systems and oxygen metabolism of the September canaries might have been badly damaged by the deadly combination of the terror and toxicity of the day.

There was no outcry among doctors for the September canaries. Who had the courage to go up against the *Journal*?

***

You are often still a mess
Though these days,
At times,
You weep because
You miss Him.

Hafiz

The Tragedy in Simple Words

The September Eleven syndrome was often considered a medical mystery. It need not have been. It was often stated that all laboratory tests were negative in the victims of the syndrome. That was not true. Doctors believed the September Eleven syndrome was not treatable. Nothing could have been further from the truth. Doctors were uneasy with the September canaries. They did not have to be.

Why were doctors so confused about the cause of the syndrome? Because it did not fit into some neat model of a specific disease in their textbooks. Why was it not treated successfully? Because there were no effective drugs for it.

In simple words, the tragedy of the September canaries was a tragedy of doctors who stubbornly refused to learn:

1. How to detect injury to immune cells and oxygen metabolism caused by cumulative toxicity;
2. How to recognize the special nutritional needs of the September canaries;
3. How to administer nutrient therapies to support the special nutritional needs of those canaries; and
4. How to use natural detox therapies to reduce the total body burden of environmental toxins.

The Poisoned People of a Poisoned City

In 2005, there were over 250,000 September canaries in the City. On a September morning four years earlier, the City had been savagely brutalized. Many lives had been lost. The destruction of the City property had neither been assessed nor understood. For days, the people could not sleep and walked around in a haze—fearful and angry at some times, confused and humiliated at others. The officials closed all tunnels and bridges in the City. All planes were forced to land, none allowed to fly out. People remained glued to their TV sets, hoping for the nightmare to end. The shops were empty, as were the restaurants. Many businesses folded.

Then something happened in the City that had never been witnessed before. The people rose to face the catastrophe in the spirit and courage expected of a truly great city. They discovered the power of the national flag. They felt united and strengthened under the flag in ways never before imagined. They spoke to strangers—not their custom in the past—to ease their pain. Concerts had been held to raise huge sums of money to help the families of those who had perished. The City leaders had spoken of resolve and steadfastness. The City will defend itself, they had proclaimed. The City will be built again, had been the resounding slogan. And so it came to pass. Spending money became a patriotic mission. By 2003, the City had risen, transcendent in splendor.

But everything did not go right. The problems of anxiety and anger persisted. Millions of people in the City and its environs experienced difficulty in falling or staying sleep. Hundreds of thousands of them developed stomach troubles, heart palpitations, and persistent tiredness. Common infections became more common, the healing processes delayed. With passing months, many people overcame their health problems. They returned to their passions —shopping, sports, and sulking.

But that was not the case with the human canaries among them—those with weak constitutions. Their abdominal symptoms worsened and they suffered headaches, sore throats, skin rashes, malaise, and body aches that did not let up. With passing months, their muscle and tissue became sensitive, and the pain and debilitation caused by their symptom-complexes triggered by the events of that September morning became continual. The sick suffered from unrelenting exhaustion, could not work, and were brain-fogged.

In 2002, the medical journals attributed the health problems to relentless anxiety. The journals considered the anxiety and sleep difficulties as symptoms of a variant of the post-traumatic stress syndrome. Antidepressants were recommended for treatment, but those drugs helped but little. The doctors were baffled and helpless. They neither understood what caused the malady nor had any remedies for it. A few physicians began to suspect deeper problems, such as ongoing injury to the immune system.

In 2002, I put forth the simple theory that the victims of the September Eleven syndrome had developed progressive cellular toxicity that resulted in a state of dysfunctional oxygen metabolism that explained all their symptoms. Most doctors, however, did not believe there was any merit to that viewpoint. Indeed, many of them found the ideas amusing.

During the months that followed, the September canaries were afflicted by a widening spectrum of unusual and progressive symptom-complexes. They began to recognize that there was something deeply wrong within them—some radical change in their bodies that fundamentally affected their energy and immune systems. They found explanations offered by their doctors superfluous, shallow and without substance. It was then that the term the September Eleven syndrome took hold.

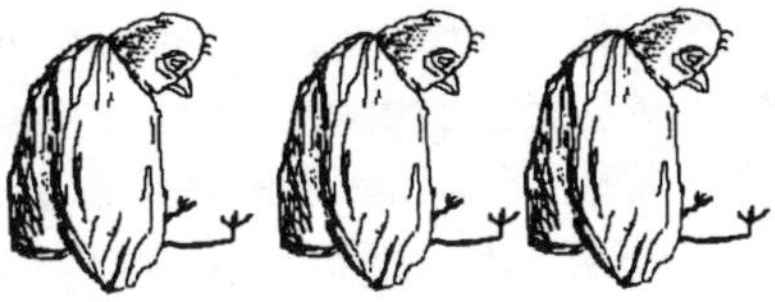

Everywhere the old order changes
and happy they who can change.

Sir William Osler.

It Doesn't Kill You,
But It Kills Who You Are

A peculiar aspect of the September Eleven syndrome was that the sick often could not describe their suffering well. When the sick women complained of severe menstrual cramps, bloating, and disturbing mood swings, their doctors nodded knowingly—so, what's new about PMS, they told themselves—and prescribed painkillers. When the ill men reported difficulties of mood, memory, and mentation, the doctors smiled condescendingly—exaggerated stress response, they told themselves—and prescribed anxiolytic drugs. But the syndrome did not let up. The hearts of the September canaries faltered. Their bowels cramped and bloated. Their joints stiffened. Their muscles ached. Some told their doctors they felt as if a truck had hit them and caused internal injury everywhere. Those descriptions of symptom-complexes made no sense to attending doctors. They had never encountered such stories. Medical textbooks were silent on the issue.

Months pass, but the victims of the syndrome did not see any signs of improvement. A tolerable day here, less late-night TV watching there, but the syndrome pursued its course relentlessly. To the victims it was clear that the syndrome was spreading throughout their bodies. They also began to recognize that their doctors simply dismissed their symptom-complexes as too nonsensical to be taken seriously—some sort of medical plethora invented by troubled minds.

One day I probed the nature of the syndrome. I told a patient that I would listen closely and without interruption to everything she might say about her case. I hoped that her own insights into her suffering might enlighten me about the nature of the disorder. She looked surprised—apparently no doctor had offered her that before—and began hesitatingly, choosing her words carefully. Some minutes later she seemed to tap into some inner voice that chattered excitedly. Several more minutes elapsed. Then she realized she was rambling without making any sense. Frustrated, she stopped and stared at me. I sat listening closely. Then she blurted, "It doesn't kill you, but it kills who you are."

The Pit

A large pit was left behind in the City following the September horror. The "Pit" terrorized the City people every day, since they were shown its pictures daily. It smoldered for months. Plumes of dark smoke arose from it and spread over the City. Those who visited it reported an insufferable stench. It was expected that all City dwellers exposed to the toxic fumes would acquire some sort of respiratory ailment. That came to pass. Those with a past history of recurrent bronchitis and asthma fared worse. The children in the City—nearly one in four of whom carried an inhaler to school prior to the September events—suffered the most. The use of steroid inhaler medications exploded. Predictably, that problem was also serious among the Pit workers. Several weeks later, the Fire Commissioner reported "uneasy breathing" among four thousand of his force who had battled the inferno of the Pit.

Incinerated Stuff Laced With Jet Fuel

Monstrous black clouds billowing out of the Pit carried enormous amounts of pulverized plastics, concrete, metals, glass, and other building materials. The particulate matter was laced with incompletely combusted jet fuel. What the toxicant load was of those billowing clouds of smoke was anybody's guess. The U.S. Environmental Protection Agency (EPA) monitored the air quality. It announced that the levels of toxic chemicals were within the established standards.

Some amazing comments were included in a written statement presented to the City Council. Below, I include one quote:

> We've tested for the presence of pollutants such as asbestos, fine particulate matter, lead, volatile organic compounds, dioxin, benzene, metals, PCBs and other chemicals and substances that could pose a threat to the public and workers at the site. Fortunately, the vast majority of our tests find levels of these contaminants that *pose no significant long-term health risks to residents, business employees and visitors beyond ground zero*. [Italics added.]

How could any person, least of all an EPA official, have made that statement? *That pose no significant long-term health risks*. What possible scientific information could the Agency have had to take such an utterly indefensible position? Had they conducted any true-to-life tests of *long-term* toxicity of those pollutants? The Agency officials were not challenged with any of those questions.

More importantly, did the Agency have any scientific data on how human canaries—persons with weak constitutions or immune systems damaged by chronic sugar overload and antibiotic abuse—would be affected by *cumulative* toxic load? And by *undetermined* quantities of poisons? Following an *undetermined* period of exposure? The officials at the Agency never bothered to raise any of those questions. The Agency scientists were silent on those issues.

Months later the story changed. The Agency conceded that when hourly measurements were considered, peaks of particulate matter were recorded that surpassed the *acceptable* levels. The Agency deftly evaded all meaningful discussion of what it proclaimed were *acceptable* standards of toxic fumes, as well as how it had arrived at those values.

The issue of chemical toxicity versus chemical sensitivity was equally relevant in this matter as well. But it created the awkward problem of how to gauge the level of sensitivity—as it had been with the Gulf War canaries. The messy subject of *acceptable* levels was never addressed.

A more important issue was the matter of *cumulative load* of toxins for a given individual. For mainstream doctors, that brought in the more knotty problem of biochemical individuality. The variability of responses to total load of toxic chemicals among different individuals meant that the doctors could not prudently apply the same standards of acceptable levels of toxins. That, of course, was the crux of the matter for human canaries—people with poor constitutions.

The Magic of PCBs: Now You See It, Now You Don't

PCBs (polychlorinatedbiphenyls) are a family of synthetic chemicals well known for their ability to cause toxicity and sensitivity problems. Chemical toxicity is a dose-related phenomena; the higher the dose, the greater the toxic effects. Chemical sensitivity is dose-independent. Some vulnerable persons develop serious health problems with minimal exposures that do not cause visible ill effects in others.

Large quantities of PCBs were used in the manufacture of electrical equipment. In 1977, the United States banned the use of PCBs after the serious health hazards of that family of chemicals were recognized. But as things go, some of those materials with PCBs found their way into the construction of the Twin Towers.

The enviroment agency tested the air samples collected from the surroundings of the Pit and reported negative test results. As in the case of asbestos, the agency explained that all PCBs were incinerated at the temperatures of 1000 degrees Celsius or above in the inferno. None was left to be detected. Remembering previous false assurances regarding asbestos, people were not reassured.

Later analysis of air from the Pit revealed the presence of PCBs. No one was surprised by that.

There were large quantities of Freon used in air conditioner units in the Twin Towers. It was known that Freon can be converted into highly toxic gases, including the dreaded nerve gas, by high temperatures. No one had bothered to undertake a serious study of such toxic gases.

On January 8, 2002, nearly four months after the inferno, a TV network channel focused on the chemical toxicity of the air in the general area of the Pit—not from the Pit itself—and had several invited guests. One woman told others that she had to abandon her apartment in the area. Whenever she returned to it for picking up her mail, she suffered severe headaches of the type she had never experienced prior to September Eleven. A man described persistent dry cough, hoarseness, sinus fullness, and headache. Those symptoms were also triggered by breathing the area air. They expressed many concerns about how the known synthetic chemicals in the Towers might have been converted to much more toxic substances by chemical reactions triggered by very high temperature.

What interested me most in that program was the response of Christie Todd Whitman—the highest person on the bureaucracy of the Environmental Protection Agency at the time—to those concerns. She flatly asserted that the air posed no health hazards to the people living in the area. What possible basis of such an outlandish statement might she have?, I wondered. Whitman was not a scientist, so her personal comments might be overlooked, but the issue there was the opinion of scientists in her agency. All chemists and environmental doctors in the TV audience must have cringed at her response, as I had. You expect denials from government officials. Usually they are more circumspect. I did not think that TV program would allay anyone's fears.

Mercury From a Million Bulbs

The Twin Towers complex had approximately one million fluorescent light bulbs that contained mercury. Incineration of those bulbs released mercury in gaseous form into the massive clouds of smoke that spread all over the City.

A few months later, some firemen tested positive for mercury. The City health officials consulted toxicologists, who showed no concern for the amounts of mercury found in the bodies of firemen. One of the firemen was not satisfied with the answer and expressed concern about the long-term brain toxicity of exposure to mercury. He was thought to be a hypochondriac.

What escaped everyone's notice was that those toxicologists were experts only in theory. They were not clinicians and had very limited direct contact with victims of acute mercury toxicity. They knew well the patterns of acute mercury toxicity, such as liver and kidney injury as well as skin rashes. They had had no experience with low-grade but progressive and insidious mercury toxicity that was expected after the Twin Towers inferno. Specifically, they had no inkling about how even small amounts of mercury can tip the balance in subjects with overworked detoxification pathways. For example, persons deficient in glutathione—the quarterback defense molecule of detoxification in the liver—were especially vulnerable to minute quantities of mercury since it had a special ability to tear apart glutathione molecules.

Integrative physicians who had diligently observed patterns of subclinical low-grade mercury toxicity were not consulted. They had repeatedly observed toxicity of mercury in dental fillings put into persons with compromised immune systems. They had also encountered cases in which rapid mercury chelation with oral and intravenous chelating agents—such as DMSA and DMPS—had resulted in obvious brain toxicity, including serious encephalitis-like symptoms in some patients. There were other subtle patterns of mercury toxicity. To cite an example, one victim of the syndrome had a delayed menstrual cycle after each of four sessions of removal of dental amalgams.

Mercury toxicity was considered a controversial issue. It need not have been. The neurotoxicity of mercury was well established. It was also known that the urine level of mercury after DMPS chelation was an excellent indicator of mercury buildup. The problem was that mainstream doctors did not perform the right test (post DMPS chelation), nor did they learn how to use oral DMSA treatment to rid the body of mercury load. It seemed convenient to disregard the blood mercury level. In essence, the mercury problem was simply pushed under the proverbial rug.

Mercury in Landfills, Mercury in Dental Fillings

Mercury was a major ingredient in many products, from thermometers and fluorescent bulbs to batteries and old latex paint. The environmentalists were very concerned about mercury vapor rising from the landfills. The dentists showed little, if any, concern about mercury toxicity caused by dental fillings.

In its August 2000 issue, *Atmosphere Environment* reported finding mercury concentrations in the open air over landfills that were deemed at least 1,000 times that of any dimethyl mercury concentration ever recorded. Dimethyl mercury, it may be pointed out here, is far more toxic than monomethyl mercury. The article went on: Sending mercury-containing waste to landfills may essentially be spoon-feeding copious amounts of the toxicant to methylating bacteria.

There was also concern about children eating fish from mercury-contaminated waters. The July 2001 issue of *Science News* carried the following quote:

> Some 60,000 US children are born each year with developmental impairments triggered by fetal exposure to methyl mercury, usually as a result of their moms having eaten tainted fish.

There was no concern expressed about mercury in amalgams in the mouths of little children, whose mothers were warned against brain toxicity from eating tainted fish.

Fresh Kills

Nearly a million tons of toxic debris from the Pit had to be taken somewhere. The City picked an area called Fresh Kills landfill as its dump. It was predictable that the dump would become a sacred ground because the debris brought to it contained human remains.

Much of the poisonous material brought to Fresh Kills gradually outgassed. The emanations from the huge site would be expected to kill wildlife. And that happened. Within months, many residents of surrounding communities experienced symptoms which their doctors could not explain. The EPA officials insisted that the poisons coming out of Fresh Kills were within *acceptable* limits and posed no health threats to anyone. That did not surprise me. EPA had a long history of downplaying the real hazards of toxic chemicals. They were not only proficient in misstating their findings, they had also become very comfortable with misinterpretations of data which suited them.

The following comment was included by the chief official of the Agency's City office in her written statement to the City Council:

> I'm sure that many of you saw the *Daily News* headlines last Friday heralding a "Toxic Zone" at ground zero. While the data in the story were accurate, the interpretation of the data and the context was not.

The interpretation of the data and the context was not! The words both amazed and saddened me. Who at the Agency decided the interpretation was not right?, I wondered. All of the Agency's toxicologists were chemists who, by law, could not care for persons with environmental illness. The Agency also retained the services of some doctors who neither cared for the sick nor practiced nutritional medicine. They had no understanding of clinical problems caused by toxic chemicals. Their primary purpose was to support EPA's interpretations of the data. They provided what was claimed to be the "outside expert opinion" by the Agency.

For decades, hundreds of the physician members of the American Academy of Environmental Medicine had diligently documented case histories of environmentally sensitive persons. They had understood the critical difference between chemical sensitivity and chemical toxicity. They had recognized the special nutritional needs of persons with environmental illness. They had also observed the clinical benefits of detox therapies. The EPA officials found much comfort in the fact that mainstream doctors—persons without an understanding of environmental sensitivity issues—had dismissed environmental physicians as quacks.

The Environmental Protection Agency had never sought the counsel of physician members of the Academy. Nor did they ever retain the services of physicians trained in environmental medicine to clinically evaluate those afflicted by environmental pollutants.

So, how did the Agency decide what was the right interpretation when the *Daily News* challenged it? That question escaped the attention of the media.

Asbestos From the Pit

Asbestos aerosols spewed out from the Pit with the smoke that arose from it for months. That was not a small matter. Many years earlier, some lawyers had joined the ranks of the newly rich by famously litigating cases of asbestos toxicity. Thus, the City people were familiar with the dreaded hazards.

The Environmental Protection Agency repeatedly assured the City people that they had carefully examined multiple samples of the fumes emanating from the Pit. And that they had found no asbestos. Asbestos, they explained, had been pulverized during the inferno. The people in the City, they counseled, need not add the fear of asbestos toxicity to their ever-growing list of miseries. People in the City had considerable difficulty accepting that. Their skepticism had a clear basis.

Some doctors in the City considered themselves the top asbestos experts in the world—that, again, was *their* opinion. They took pains to explain to the public what they considered to be the critical difference between microscopic fragments of asbestos and its ultramicroscopic aerosols. Then they claimed that, with their superior technology, they had indeed found the asbestos ultraparticles not detected by the Agency officials. Next came even more frightening words: "Smaller the particle, the more easily it can be aerosolized. And the easier job that it has penetrating right down into the depths of the lung," an expert pronounced.

The war between the Agency officials and the asbestos experts lasted for months. The fears of asbestos toxicity lasted for years.

Chemical Toxicity Versus Chemical Sensitivity

Chemical toxicity is dose-dependent—the greater the amount of toxins, the greater the degree of cellular injury. Chemical sensitivity, by contrast, is dose-independent. Very small quantities of certain toxins can cause serious health problems for the sensitive individuals, but not others without specific sensitivity.

A handful of environmental doctors in the City had known the difference between the two phenomena for decades. The mainstream doctors had rejected the idea for an equally long period.

Most September canaries exhibited the classical pattern of sensitivity as their symptom-complexes became more intense. Most of them suffered from headaches and lightheadedness when they were exposed to strong perfumes, paints, cleaning solutions, formaldehyde, and tobacco smoke. Most of them also became intolerant to an increasing number of foods. The mainstream doctors dismissed those symptoms as all-in-the-head problems. The environmental doctors knew that those sensitivities were real, since they mostly cleared up when such persons were vigorously treated in the early stages of their illness.

The sicker the September canaries became, the larger the number of environmental intolerances they developed.

Anthrax: An Epidemic of Fear

Some in the City thought the cause of the Malady was *Bacillus anthracis*. I did not think so.

There were some deaths from anthrax infections. The people soon learned that anthrax infections had not been encountered in the country for decades. The possibility of a spreading fatal infection itself became an epidemic of paralyzing fear. There seemed to be no end to bad news.

People were warned that the inhaled form of anthrax infection begins like a common cold, then rapidly turns into pneumonia. Potent anthrax toxins rapidly spread throughout the body, causing high fevers, coma, and death. The folks on radio and TV saw to it that every man, woman, and child in the City was kept fully informed—and fearful.

Antibiotics were freely dispensed for the fearful. Antibiotics are designer killer molecules that draw little distinction between the disease-causing and disease-preventing microbes. The fearful were told about that hazard, but they insisted that they take the drugs. Then yet a new fear arose: It was predicted that available inventory of the antibiotic of choice for anthrax infection was not enough to provide for everyone in the case of an epidemic. The drug-maker geared up the production. Yet, the fear of the fearful persisted.

The anthrax epidemic never arrived. Antibiotic toxicity did occur. More significantly, what followed was ongoing disruption of the bowel ecosystems of the human canaries who took antibiotics.

Fear Fans Its Own Fires

It was a confusing time. The flames of the fear epidemic were fanned from the top—the President, in the words of a journalist, officially invited the country to both buck up and freak out. The Vice President was sneaked around by his guards as if he were in the witness protection program. The Congress closed its great halls. The homeland security officials warned the country against more attacks on the nation's bridges and airports. The FBI chose "skyfall" as its code word for warning citizens of imminent attack. The reporters became newsmakers. TV network and newspaper buildings were cordoned. People swarmed around the police barricades, curious and afraid.

Two hundred eighty million people in the country were exhorted to become investigators and report everything unusual or alarming in their neighborhood. People rose to the challenge and spied on their neighbors. Some reported catering trucks parked on the city streets to authorities. Others reported powdery substances on their keyboards after they ate cookies over them. So many school buildings were evacuated that one governer posted a reward of $10,000 for arrests of hoaxers in his state.

Many couples rushed for marriage licenses. A larger number called divorce lawyers. People reviewed their wills and then tucked them away. Fathers wanted to reassure their children. They told them there were greater chances of their getting killed in traffic when moms were on cell phones than by the acts of terrorists. Psychiatrists thrived on dissection of what they believed was the pathology of fear.

Sleepless in the City

For the citizens, restless sleep was a particularly distressing symptom during weeks and months after the September events. The anxiety about not being able to sleep further compounded the problem. The City had the best doctors anywhere—that, of course, was *their* opinion. Though puzzled by the malady, many of them rose to the occasion to heal the City. They ministered to the needs of the sick with empathy and diligence that touched their patients deeply. They obligingly handed out scripts for sleeping and anxiety pills. Next, they conducted complex studies of the disturbed sleep patterns of the September canaries with their Star Wars medical technology and diligently classified the sleep disorders they "discovered." Then they prescribed sleep machines. When that did not work, they administered antidepressants.

Sleep was also threatened by severe cases of media-*itis*. There were blizzards of 'network news' that kept the people alive until late night hours. There were scares about infectious epidemics that did not arrive. Experts on many channels worked hard to keep the audience informed about all kinds of possible attacks on them by unseen enemies. There was talk about the possibility of nuclear holocaust. The people remained edgy and sleepless.

There were yet other threats to sleep. The rich in the City had many fears. They saw their fortunes being wiped out. Indeed, before the sick had thought of the term September Eleven syndrome, the money managers had used it in their cries of despair. They understood the cost of closed airports, tunnels, and bridges. They recognized what would happen if the people did not return to shops and restaurants very soon. Consumer confidence— they knew only too well—is what drives the economy. They knew they needed help from the Congress. They also understood that some suitable slogan—some powerful buzzword, to be precise—was required to move the Congress. The treasury doors were hard to pry open. Ever so ingenious, the money managers coined the syndrome and used it deftly and profitably. But the efforts to goad the Congress required vigorous radio and TV ad campaigns. Some chilling predictions of impending collapse of the national economy had to be made—repeatedly and continually. That wreaked havoc on the frayed nerves of the citizens and further deepened the sleep problems.

Within months, a scientific study and an editorial in the leading medical journal sized up the problem accurately. Forty-four percent of the people in the *country* had suffered one or more substantial stress symptoms. One-fourth of them had trouble falling or staying asleep. It was easy to gather statistics about the incidence of sleep disorders. Restoring the sleep of the afflicted was another matter.

I recognized an evolving and sinister clinical pattern. I knew that the sleep difficulties portended the development of other chronic intractable disorders. Chronic sleeplessness leads to energy dysequilibrium in the body which, in turn, sets the stage for indolent immune dysfunctions. My Gulf War canaries had given me some sense of what it meant to be a human canary. The City doctors, however, had little interest in the sleep-energy-immune dynamics.

Terror to ASD to PTSD to Psychiatric Disorder

Within minutes of the terror of the Twin Towers inferno, psychologists and psychiatrists predicted that millions of people in the City would suffer from acute stress disorder (ASD). Within hours, the talk turned from ASD to post-traumatic stress disorder (PTSD). Four months later, in its January 10, 2002, issue, the *New England Journal of Medicine* advised its readers that PTSD was the fourth most common psychiatric disorder in the country.

The *Journal*, of course, was the most powerful voice in medicine in the country. No one was expected to challenge it when it labeled the biologic effects of the terror and toxicity of unremitting stress as psychiatric illness. And none did.

The *Journal* told its readers that well over 100,000 people directly witnessed the events of September Eleven and, based on the Oklahoma experience, predicted that over 35,000 persons in the City will develop post-traumatic stress disorder—the first such epidemic of psychiatric disorder anywhere in the history of the world.

Huge masses of people in Manhattan, Brooklyn, and New Jersey had directly witnessed the collapse of the Twin Towers. The *Journal* did not state how it managed to reduce their numbers to 100,000. More curious to me was its disregard of the much larger number of people who were brutalized by the TV screens everywhere.

Beyond the minor issue of meaningless numbers published by the *Journal* was the grievous mistake of giving the diagnosis of psychiatric illness to those hurt by the terror and toxicity of the September events. There was not one word about how the poisons from the Pit might have poisoned the victims. Not one word about the cellular toxicity caused by those poisons. Not one word about the damaged energy and detoxification pathways of people exposed to those poisons. Not one word about immune injury.

The City doctors joined psychologists and psychiatrists in recognizing the need for aggressive psychologic interventions to prevent the development of delayed and intractable chronic syndromes triggered and perpetuated by unremitting fear and stress.

The *Journal* authoritatively turned biologic toxicity into psychiatric illness. The September canaries had to further suffer the indignity of being considered mentally imbalanced.

You do not bite the hand that feeds you, I had heard a long time ago. The *Journal* was evidently wise about such matters. The real issues of too much oxidation and not enough oxygen could not be effectively addressed by drugs. That was the turf of integrative medicine. There was no drug money there. Why offend its rich friends in the pharmaceutical and insurance industries?

Fear and Anxiety? Yes.
Immune Injury and Oxygen Dysfunction? No.

In 2002, when the September canaries presented with recurrent infections with delayed healing—to them a clear sign of immune weakness—their doctors expressed doubts that such infections had anything to do with the September events. They prescribed antibiotics, which rarely helped. They ordered tests for low-grade ongoing inflammation—C-reactive and other types of proteins—and frequently found those tests to be positive. But they did not know what to make of those test results in the absence of clinical signs of acute or chronic inflammation. They also used batteries of tests for immune dysfunctions, which usually came back negative, except for the test for antinuclear antibodies (ANA) that was commonly positive. Again, they were frustrated because the textbook models of immune diseases could not be diagnosed only by positive ANA test results, nor by positive tests for low-grade inflammatory response anywhere in the body. They thought they had no choice except to wait for the disorder to differentiate with time sufficiently to become diagnosable.

Sometimes doctors were candid and told the September canaries about their wait-and-see strategy. The logic of their position exasperated the canaries. "My doctor wants to wait until my disease becomes advanced enough for him to diagnose," a September canary once told me. The true nature of their suffering—immune dysfunction caused by *cumulative* toxicity of events of that September— escaped them simply because they did not ask the right questions nor did they look in the right places for the answers. The issues of cellular toxicity and dysfunctional oxygen metabolism were ignored.

In 2003, when the September canaries complained of persistent air hunger and brain fog—to them clear signs of oxygen dysfunction—their doctors ordered batteries of tests to find out if there were problems of the heart and lungs. They found none. Tests for anemia were also negative. However, the doctors neglected to order tests that would have revealed the presence of dysfunctional oxygen metabolism at a cellular level. All September canaries showed a heavy buildup of toxic organic acids in their bodies, such as citric acid, fumaric acid, succinic acid, lactic acid, and related acids. The increased excretion of those acids in 24-hour urine samples was undeniable evidence of cellular oxygen dysfunction. However, it was not the practice to perform those tests in the City hospitals. What tests were not done at hospitals had little, if any, interest for the City doctors. They were not interested in wrestling with the complexities of the terror and toxicity of the Twin Towers.

Terror Turns Into Toxicity, Toxicity Into Terror

I never understood how psychologists separate the mind from the body, and medical doctors the body from the mind. To be candid, I found their theories silly and irrelevant to my clinical work. Clearly, those theories had no scientific merit. My view on the subject was reinforced by many September canaries. Their bodies and minds spoke eloquently of how the terror of the Twin Towers inferno turned into toxicity, and its toxicity into terror. It puzzled me why the City doctors did not see the obvious that the September canaries described so succinctly. For years after the September events, the City doctors continued to insist that the victims of the September Eleven syndrome suffered from the post-traumatic stress syndrome—they had declared that syndrome to be a psychiatric disorder decades earlier—but that there was no evidence that they also suffered from serious immune dysfunction.

The First Psychiatric Epidemic

So it came to pass that the City witnessed its first psychiatric epidemic—a black malady that affected more than a quarter of million people. Indeed, it was the first time the world had known an epidemic of psychiatric disease of that magnitude.

Within a year the doctors in the City had lost interest in that epidemic. The City had the most gifted epidemiologists anywhere—that, again, was their opinion of themselves—who had doggedly investigated other epidemics in the City for decades until they claimed to have unravelled the full mystery of those afflictions. I never understood why the greatest of all epidemics ever to hit the City escaped their enormous investigative talent.

Should Not Overly Medicalize Them

Perhaps the reason for the City epidemiologist losing interest in the great psychiatric epidemic were the article published in *The New England Journal of Medicine.* In its Febuary 21, 2002 issue (page 629), the *Journal* had the following to say in two pieces about the victims of the September Eleven syndrome:

> Although the events of September 11 were profoundly traumatic for those directly involved and clearly distressing for others, they are *not necessarily medically significant*. [italic added].

Then the *Journal* gave its counsel in simple words:

> Although we should acknowledge our natural emotional reactions to tragic events, we *should not overly medicalize them*. [Italics added].

Our emotional reactions! The *Journal* here is clearly concerned about the emotional reactions of its readers—the physicians, including the epidemiologists. The advice about not medicalizing concerned the victims. The *Journal* went on:

> We anticipate that a subgroup of people might have a harder time recovering, because they were directly exposed to the attacks or because of their personal characteristics (e.g., a history of mental health problem).

Every onee knew that the *Journal* spoke the truth. And that only the folks on the fringe were foolish enough to go up against it.

I Thought I'd Be Over it by Now

The position taken by *The New England Journal of Medicine* troubled me much for another reason. It was at a marked variance with what the City media was reported continuously. For example, the March 18, 2002 issue of *New York* magazine ran a cover story about the unprecendented number of New Yorkers who continued to suffer from debilitating nightmares, psychosomatic illnesses, marital troubles, and depression. The magazine expressed great concern over the activities at the City's crisis hotline. The agency received distress calls with increasing frequency such that an astonishing 6,600 people reached for their phones on January 1, 2002. Before September 11, the average number of daily calls was near one hundred. Consider the following quote from *New York:*

> The initial numbness that followed September 11 may have worn off, but the seismic shock to the city's collective psyche is still producing new and surprising symptoms.... What happened here, which is extremely rare, is that people who weren't anywhere near the Trade towers are developing traumatic reactions....What I hear over and over again is the same thing: 'I thought I'd be over it by now.'

I did not think that the authorities at *The New England Journal of Medicine* were going to be impressed by reports like the one cited above from *New York.* And they were not.

Banalities of Gurus of Celebrity Medicine

The media did take interest in the subject of the terror and toxicity of the September events. They invited some well-known medical writers to come and explain the public health issues arising from the September conflagration. They came up with banalities which passed as expert medical opinion. I did not think their frivolous notions of post-traumatic stress disorder were going to help anyone who had become a September canary.

It escaped the notice of the media that those celebrities had become medical celebrities not because they had any passion for the sick. Rather, they had a passion for the art of becoming a celebrity. They rarely, if ever, cared for the sick.

That is what had happened years earlier with the Gulf War canaries. Their pain and suffering were countered with banalities from medical celebrities. The September canary sufferers just simply followed their footsteps.

Millions for Drugs, Nothing for Nutrients and Detoxicants

Enormous sums of money were raised by private philanthropic efforts to help those afflicted by the September events. A substantial portion of those funds were allocated for the medical needs of the victims. The government offered additional funds as medical grants.

I knew that every dollar of those monies would be snatched up by doctors who knew how to play well the grant money game. Every dollar would be spent in looking at the plight of the September canaries with the prevailing one-toxin/one-disease/one-drug models of medical research. I predicted that nothing of real clinical value would come out of those studies—as had been the case with the Gulf War canaries. *When a population is affected by dozens of poisons, a focus on only one of those poisons does not reveal the true story of chemical toxicity and sensitivity in those people.*

I was not surprised. No funds were allocated to see how vigorous integrative programs of nutrient support, chemical detoxification, and spiritual support could restore the health of those tormented by the terror and toxicity of the time. Some small groups of the September canaries tried to take an activist role to secure funding for that purpose. They were no more successful than the Gulf War canaries had been before them. Their voices were drowned in the loud music of men of money in medicine. When they persisted, they were condescendingly told that the methods they were advocating were not scientific. The science of causing toxicity with drugs was acceptable, that of detoxification with nutrients was not. Clinical nutrition had never been deemed a proper field of inquiry by those who held the purse strings of the medical research money.

Betty Best, M.D., Anita Average, M.D., and the September Eleven Syndrome

Several months after September Eleventh, I knew of two practitioners in the City who committed their full energies to the treatment of the September Eleven syndrome. One of them, Betty Best, M.D., a highly esteemed university internist, took a strongly academic approach to the problem. She ordered many laboratory tests and scans to make precise diagnoses and diligently recorded all findings concerning her patients' illness. She planned to author a definitive book about the syndrome. The second physician was Anita Average, M.D. She practiced holistic medicine and ordered only a limited number of diagnostic tests.

I recognized a highly unusual opportunity to examine the syndrome. I proposed that the National Institutes of Health in Washington, D.C., conduct a clinical trial of remarkable simplicity. I suggested that two hundred city firemen with symptom-complexes that developed after September Eleven be included in the study. Alphabetically, the first hundred be assigned to Betty Best, M.D. and the second hundred be given to Anita Average, M.D. Both Drs. Best and Average will be given full authority to order any tests and prescribe any therapies, without any regard to the cost of testing or treatment.

I knew Anita Average was no match for Betty Best in designing, conducting, and publishing a clinical trial. Betty Best had an amazing grasp of the prevailing disease classifications. She was also a mesmerizing speaker. By contrast, poor Anita Average was clumsy with her descriptions of what she thought ailed her patients. She was incapable of using powerful and complex data analysis models which Betty Best was best at. It was clear to me that Dr. Best would prescribe the best available drug therapies—essentially a blockade medicine with drugs that suppress neurotransmitters, block cell receptors and channels, and inhibit cell enzymes and pumps. She would most likely ask for psychiatric consultations for many of her patients. Anita Average, on the other hand, would choose supportive nutrient and herbal therapies, with a serious effort to involve her patients with spiritual work to cope with pain and anguish caused by the syndrome.

I surmised that there would be no point bringing Betty Best and Anita Average together for the clinical trial. Indeed, I suspected that Betty Best would not even agree to doing the study if she found out that her results would be compared with those of Anita Average. I did not anticipate the possibility of any debates between the two doctors. So, I proposed that the trial be continued for three years, without either knowing what the other was being asked to do. More importantly, at the end of three years, the sick themselves would be allowed to assess the benefits of the two different approaches. Specifically, the sufferers of the September Eleven syndrome would be asked to assess the quality of their: (1) general energy level; (2) physical fitness; (3) sleep; (4) digestion and bowel health; (5) mood, memory and mentation; (6) capacity for work; and (7) the ability to live, learn, laugh, and love.

I thought such a clinical trial would yield two important insights into the September Eleven syndrome: First, how does the combination of holistic therapies with spiritual work stack up against the treatment plan of synthetic drugs and psychiatric support; and Second, the victims of the syndrome could then choose the superior plan. I felt confident that the difference between three years of blockade medicine and supportive holistic therapies—as assessed and scored by the sick themselves—would be clear. Regrettably, the folks at NIH were not interested in my proposal. Indeed, they thought I was a good comedian.

Part 2

A description of the many faces of the syndrome.

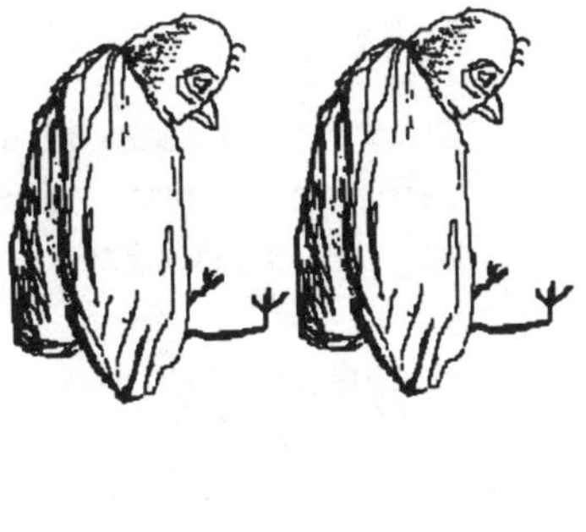

Air Hunger of the September Canaries

The September Eleven syndrome had yet other evil faces. One of the most troublesome symptoms experienced by its victims was air hunger. That description exasperated their doctors. The cardiologists performed cardiograms, echocardiograms, and heart scans, and pronounced the heart to be normal. They often noted some racing of the heart, which they readily attributed to anxiety. The pulmonologists analyzed blood gases and found normal oxygen saturation levels. Lung scans were read as negative by radiologists. The hematologists ran tests for anemia, but found none. How could anyone with a healthy heart, lungs, and blood *ever* be hungry for air?, they asked in frustration.

And yet, the victims of the syndrome continued to report air hunger. They used words to express their sensations which would be hard for anyone to make up. Here is how many human canaries struggled to put their anguish in words:

- I'm breathing, but I'm not.
- How can I be so short-winded when I do so little?
- I'm only nineteen, but I breathe like I were a ninety-one-year-old. That's what this September syndrome has done to me.
- I'm oxygen-starved. Has anyone ever told you that? I mean, can someone who doesn't have pneumonia or heart attack get oxygen-starved?
- Breathing takes so much energy. I feel silly saying that.

- It's like someone cut my air by one-half.

- It's oxygen. I know I don't have enough of it. I just know that.

- I have the metabolism of a snake. I don't really know what that is. I guess what I'm saying is that there is not much air in me.

- I work 20 hours a week in an antique shop. It is a lot of fun. But sometimes I can't breathe there. I have this air hunger, then my chest hurts.

- After three dances, my muscles suddenly went dead. I simply couldn't breathe, just like they tell you what happens after a heart attack.

The doctors were annoyed by such descriptions of the symptoms which they could neither understand nor treat. But they learned to ignore it. Many patients and several months later, some of them began to wonder if the frequent complaint of air hunger was, in reality, a variant of the obsessive-compulsive disorder (OCD). In that scenario, a person with OCD was clued about the frivolous notion of air hunger by a nonsensical comment of someone else. Then the neurochemistry of that disorder took over. The hunger became the new focus of OCD impulses. The more a victim of the September Eleven syndrome insisted that the symptom of air hunger was real, the surer the doctor became of the correctness of his diagnosis of OCD. That, of course, was not the first time the label of OCD poured salt on the wounds of the sick.

Then This September Thing Struck and I Have Never Been the Same

- I feel my body is toxic. My muscles are contaminated. I work out to get rid of the toxins. That flushes the stuff out, but then it all comes back. I'm 39 years old. Two years ago I had such energy, was so full of life. Then this September thing struck and I have never been the same. I was in such pain I said I would do anything to get rid of that. I agreed to have neck surgery. Several days later, my orthopedic surgeon looked at my wound and said,

  "Hey, that's great! The wound is healed."
  "But I haven't," the words slipped out.

- This thing has knocked me for a loop. I don't even remember 2002 and 2003.

- Closing the eyes without closing the eyes...it is still the mind.

- My brain is shutting down. There is nothing there. After seeing six MDs, I thought my life was over.

- You forget how you thought normally. Now, does that make sense?

The Tale of a Pediatric September Canary Told by Her Mom

Our pediatrician saw her. I told him she was tired all the time. He said, "It is chronic fatigue syndrome, but I don't want to label it that way because she is too young for it." I told his associate she sleeps all the time. She replied, "Take it from me. I'm a mother. She will get better when she grows up." I consulted a third pediatrician who said, "She is making herself sick. You should take her to a psychiatrist." The fourth pediatrician diagnosed chronic fatigue and said that it is something she will have to deal with. A neurologist ordered a tilt test that turned out to be positive. She had blurred vision and couldn't read, she often passed out. She was treated with antibiotics for six months for Lyme disease, even though the tests were negative. Antibiotics helped the first time. She used antibiotics again for one month. A pediatric cardiologist repeated the tilt test which was positive again. She took Florinef for six months. That helped her dizziness but her other symptoms worsened. A psychiatrist prescribed Zoloft. A gastroenterologist performed endoscopy and said the inside of the stomach was red in some places. Nothing else. A cardiologist diagnosed a slight case of mitral valve prolapse. Migraine headaches did not let her talk to her friend on the phone. Her face often broke out with rashes. She got fever blisters without any reason. She had low-grade fevers that remained unexplained. Hot and cold flashes trouble her. Once she missed more than 40 days of school. Naturally, her grades fell. Sore throats did not let up. Once she collapsed at her aunt's house. Her father had to carry her out. Now, four pediatricians, two gastroenterologists, two neurologists, one cardiologist, and one infectious disease specialist later, we still do not have any answers to what makes her sick. Nor are we given any clear hope of recovery.

Now I'm Simply Mad

The following is a story of an adult September canary in her own words:

When I was a child I remember having colds and sore throats all the time. I lived on antibiotics and throat lozenges. Tonsillectomy and removal of adenoids helped for some time. Then sore throats returned. I grew up and learned about yeast infections. A naturopath said that was the result of excessive antibiotics. Later, my mouth and eyes were dry. My doctor diagnosed Sjögren's syndrome. I asked, where did that come from? He shrugged. Then came osteochondritis, tingling and numbness, like electrical currents in my head, back and arms. I had heart palpitations and tightness in my chest. A cardiologist checked me and told me my heart was okay. He said that all my problems were due to stress. I knew I had allergies in my childhood, but then they returned with a vengeance. I was allergic to everything under the sun. Then came muscle pain and pain everywhere. You touch me anywhere and it hurts.

Then problems with dry eyes, dry mouth and dry nose worsened. In 2002, high stress and, I guess, fear of September events brought on chest symptoms. A rheumatologist diagnosed fibromyalgia, a second one confirmed the diagnosis. Then I got depressed and was given Prozac. No one in my family has serious depression. My husband is supportive, but this thing put severe stress on my relationship with my husband. Then new symptoms appeared, including burning in my head, severe fatigue, and pain everywhere. I couldn't sleep. I basically stayed in my bed all the time. My abdomen was bloated. I had this tremendous fire in my head. It was like living with my head in an oven. My face had all these rashes. I had trigger points everywhere. Walking on a small incline exhausted me. I lost all my sex drive. Emotionally, I was so brittle.

My whole life revolved around trying to not get any worse. My chiropractor tells me it is yeast in the head. My family doctor laughed at that diagnosis. He sent me to a neurologist. He found nothing wrong with me. MRI and CAT scans were negative. I saw two other neurologists. They told me the same thing. They found nothing wrong with me as well. The last neurologist I saw referred me to a psychiatrist who told me I was depressed and prescribed Zoloft. I didn't think I was depressed. Yes, I was depressed, but who in my shoes would not be depressed? Now I don't think I am depressed. Now I'm simply mad. I am mad because it has been three years and I am getting worse.

Waiting for Godot!

The prevailing definition of September eleventh syndrome was eminently suited to those who believed drugs were the only legitimate therapies for all diseases. They were quite clear in their heads.

They had named the syndrome. That meant they understand the problem. That also meant that all that was then required was for some drug company to come up with a drug to cure that dreadful syndrome. Waiting for another triumph of synthetic chemistry! Waiting for another miracle drug! Waiting for Godot!

What I Miss Most Is My Mind

Another distressing symptom of the syndrome was brain fog. That perplexed the doctors to no end. They ran MRI brain scans and found them to be within normal limits. The PET scans demonstrated diminished blood supply to certain parts of the brain, which they attributed to anxiety and the stress syndrome. But the enigma of brain fog remained unresolved. The medical texts and journals were silent on the issue. Some open-minded doctors had offered an interesting explanation for brain fog. The problems of mood, memory, and mentation in the Malady, they cautioned, were caused by cumulative cellular toxicity in the brain. But that was not taken seriously by the main body of doctors.

Here is how some September canaries described their brain fog:

- I'll have a discussion, but I will not remember what the conversation was all about. That is what the September Malady has done to me.
- I know what I need to do, but all I get from my brain are echoes. It is worst with numbers. I was so good at that.
- I get this mind lock and then I can't think anymore.
- I walk like a drunk, running into my door jamb, like I have had a stroke.
- I spend hours looking at same files over and over again. Sometimes I have to read the same sentence several times.

Now an attorney can't afford that, can he?

- I was a voracious reader. Now, with this thing I can't read anymore. Hard to believe, isn't it?

- Something slithers down my throat and I get woozy.

- My thinking has slowed down. It's like some moth eating my brain from inside.
- I get so adrenalized it becomes paralyzing.

- I don't focus on anything anymore. You know, it doesn't seem to matter anymore.

- I'm dizzy thinking until the basic stuff becomes impossible.

- It's like carbonation in my head. You know what I mean, don't you? Like bubbles in my head. It all started when I suddenly became sick in the plane. Then I realized my plane was on the ground. It was frightening. It still is. I can't think. My work is conceptual. Do you know how frightening that is, not to think?

Maybe I Need a Lobotomy

- I'm afraid, but don't know of what. Strange, isn't it? See what this September thing has done to me.

- I want to forget about it. Every time I think of it, I get sick.

- No, I don't think much these days. Thinking simply takes too much energy.

- It is as if English is my second language. I forget simple words like garage. Would you believe the other day I wondered about the room where my car sleeps?

- My doctor told me it was all in my head, but I'm sure glad it shows up some place. (A physician-canary's words when shown damaged cells and microclots in his blood smears.)

- One silly thought and it's like a can of worms, thoughts come out like worms. There is no end, the same thing over and over again. It was never like that.

- So, what do I do? Do I have to go back to my mother's womb, get my genes rearranged, and then return to this world all fixed, is that it?

- I was mostly a grade A student. I'm so messed up. Now simple words confuse me. Maybe I need a lobotomy.

I Fight Him in My Dreams

- My husband was very disorganized, but we never fought during the 48 years we were together. He has been gone for four years. I never quarreled with him in dreams. Since the September mess, I fight him in my dreams.

- It is as if I'm an arm's length from darkness, this dense thing...that I am going to fall into it and never get out of it. I used to be free of pain in my dreams, now I hurt in my dreams.

- My daughter called me at work and said, "Mom, I thought I'll read you what I read in my psychology book today. It says chronic myalgia is all psychological." I put the phone down and wanted to cry.

- It's like somebody beat me on my arms and legs with a baseball bat.

- I'm a broken doll.

- Very difficult to tell whether it is muscle pain or skin pain.

- I used to think I could control the muscle pain with a lot of stretching. Now I know that's silly. This thing simply does not let me sleep unless I take ibuprofen.

- Out of the blue, I get hit with a truck. That's the end of everything. Do other patients with fibromyalgia tell you that also?

- The pain used to be constant, now sometimes it fades away, then returns crashing, to my collar areas, then to my shoulders, then all over. Then I think with utter certainty that it will never go away.

- Many people with this thing tell me they have painful trigger points in their muscles. Some pain! It isn't like any pain I ever had and I always thought I had a high pain threshold. This is a killer...and it's a killer at all times.

- When it rains, an elephant sits on me.

- I walk ten minutes and it is as if I have hit a wall, like I have spent the whole day's energy.

- I have can't-get-out-of-my-bed syndrome. (A September canary's self-diagnosis.)

- I sleep better when I pass out. I become dizzy thinking, then basic stuff becomes hard, like do blue socks go with a green shirt? Ridiculous, isn't it? Then my mind races. I think too much of everything. Like taking a shower, personal hygiene. I know several languages, now I tire just thinking of words. Maybe I shouldn't shave because I might cut myself, I tell myself, then get disgusted with myself.... even something as basic as going to the bathroom. I'm always in a hyper drive. I don't mind mood swings, I just want to be able to turn them on and off. Some things I said at work were misunderstood. Sometimes I thought I was the subject of some social experimentation.

Depression

- I'm depressed because my body is changing. Many things are happening. No one has an answer.

- I got to a level where I was feeling dead, but not suicidal.

- The main reason I could give up amitriptyline was my control of sugar.

  (The relationship between sugar blues caused by addictive consumption of sugar and depressive thoughts was not recognized by many psychiatrists, who prescribed antidepressant rather than give proper nutritional advice to victims of the Malady.)

- When I'm not well, I have this unexplained sadness, that leads to depression. It troubles me to listen to normal people tell me what they do. When I feel better, I laugh at myself.

- I was always a happy, active child. Now I'm a teenager, mostly staying in my bed, frustrated, and weepy. My friends think it's strange I'm not depressed, only weepy. I was at the top of my class, now it is so much harder to take my exams. I still know the answers but I need much more time...like my thinking has slowed down.

Hypochondria: A Cruel Word Used by Doctors to Pour Salt on the Wounds of the Sick.

A female canary once spoke bitterly of how her doctor had condescendingly dismissed her complaints because he thought she was a hypochondriac. I asked her what she thought hypochondria might be. She replied, "Hypochondria is a cruel word used by doctors to pour salt on the wounds of the sick." Following are some other canary thoughts on the subject:

- If you don't want to suffer any more than you're suffering, don't tell anyone.
- Why should I pretend to be sick to get more attention when I get a lot more attention when I am well?
- My doctor makes me feel I'm a bouquet of diseases.
- My doctor gets annoyed when I ask questions! He thinks I'm fit like a fiddle. Once he told me I'm much better at asking questions than he is at answering them.
- My doctor told me we had to wait. For what? He said, "We need to wait until this problem can differentiate itself." I guess he wants to wait until I'm much sicker and he can make some elegant diagnosis.
- My doctor thinks I'm a hypochondriac...because he says all my lab test results are negative. Do you want to know what I think of that?Hypochondria is a wicked word used by ignorant insensitive doctors to pour salt on the wounds of the suffering.

- Hypochondria is when I'm suffering and my doctor can't find the reason. If a doctor tells me there is nothing wrong with me, I get frightened, then I think I'm a hypochondriac.

- When my doctor implies I'm a hypochondriac, it's so hard not to wish this illness on him.

Children With Vast Power Over the Sick

- My illness it became a revelation of how the medical doctors in our country operate, as well as government agencies. Up to now I thought they presented a united front against. Now I realize they act and react like spoiled children when they are threatened in their positions...but they are children with vast powers over the sick of our country.

Sleeping With Alligators in September

- It's like I rest in my bed with alligators all night.
- I don't fear going to bed anymore.
- I sleep like a baby. I wake up every hour and cry a little.
- I'm never ten minutes away from a nap.

I Don't Know if the Baby Will Be Safe in Me

- I have been denuded. I have no uterus, no ovaries, no breasts.

- My doctor loves steroids. I wish he would love his patients that much.

- You told me I needed less. I have finally realized you were right. I do better when I do less therapies.

- Do I want a baby? I don't know if the baby will be safe in my body. My hormones are so messed up.

I Didn't Know My Bowel Existed

- I told myself if I can't kill those parasites, I will kill myself.

- Before I became sick, things were different. All my life I didn't know my intestine existed.

- I know it isn't real, but it feels like I haven't moved my bowels in a year.

Too Tired To Palpitate

- If I am not careful, I become lightheaded when I leave my bed.

- I had a heart attack and a stent was put in. So why am I smiling? Because I'm glad I had a heart attack rather than fibromyalgia.

- No, I don't get heart palpitations now. Maybe your protein powders helped. Or maybe my heart is too tired to palpitate now.

- I get this elevator thing. What's that? Falling free. Even water from the shower gives me tingles.

The Desert in the Eyes

- Can you do something about this sand in my eyes? I mean my eyes are always dry.
- It started with dry skin, the dry mouth, and now it's in my eyes.
- Vacancy of eyes.
- In biology class, looking through the microscope, it hurts my eyes.
- A physician asked me how my eyes were because many people with this malady have dry eyes. I replied, Dry eyes? There is a desert in my eyes!

Building the Immune System? That's Silly!

- My rheumatologist doesn't think anything is wrong with steroids, although I know steroids depress the immune system. I asked him about building up my immune system and he thought that was silly.

I Wish I Could Live in a Bubble

- I'm so afraid. I wish this thing had no name. I wish I didn't know about it. I didn't know it can be spread. I see my whole life being consumed by this thing.
- If only I could live in a bubble, I think I could get better. Things just keep hitting me, nerves and stuff!
- If only I could live in a bubble, free of other people's germs.

The September and the Spiritual

Many September canaries suffered their torments with amazing grace. Often their words touched me deeply. Following are some examples:

- Physically I'm devastated. I don't understand how I can be spiritually uplifted.
- I resented the fact that I was getting old, that I'm depressed, that I needed Prozac. Now I feel better than I have in years. Something profound is happening. I'm beginning to see the origin of the need for sugar, a sense of being centered that I have not felt for years. (From an English professor.)
- Do I pray? Yes, I do talk to Him. But for me it isn't enough.
- Do I pray? With this thing I am praying 24 hours a day.
- I see images of a strong light holding me tight and taking me through a healing path.
- I was a machine.The pain and misery of this September syndrome has turned me into a human.
- God is energy, then one should get more energy the closer one gets to Him, shouldn't one?
- My past has been painful. My present stills get rough. But my long-term prognosis is promising. I *know* that.

- Your personality gets knotted up with this September thing. When finally you do unknot it, there is more to life. You know that life becomes much larger.

- I read that serious chronic illness makes you a stronger person if it doesn't kill you first. That is so true of this malady.

- I can see some difference. I'm a thirsty person now. I don't mean in the physical sense. I guess because my cells are coming alive.

- You are too small a man and your work is too large. So here is what I tell you: keep looking up for guidance.

The Doctors' Way

- I told my doctors that my colon was bloated and the spasm of the bowel had something to do with my esophageal reflux. They smiled condescendingly and told me that wasn't the way things worked. I guess they think the stomach lives on one planet and the colon on another!

The September Canaries at Famous Clinics

The Malady had many other faces. I show some of them in quotes and bits of conversations with my patients. The voices on the following pages belong to them.

Most September canaries were intelligent people who worked regularly when they were struck with the Malady. They were neither malingerers nor hypochondriacs. They did not suffer from any mental or psychological disorders. They spoke in a matter-of-fact way that was both illuminating and compelling.

Many of those September canaries went to famous clinics in the country. After extensive tests they were told they did suffer from some strange syndrome and all that could be done for them was symptom suppression in the hope that they might get better on their own. Then they were given prescriptions for painkillers, antidepressants, and sleeping pills. As for many others, after many tests they were told there was really nothing wrong with them and all that they needed was some psychotherapy.

Pay for Poisons, But Not for Nutrients

There was another enigma concerning the September syndrome. The doctors were willing to try all possible drug therapies for its victims but they vehemently denounced the use of nutrient therapies by a handful of integrative physicians.

- My doctors pumped a lot of antibiotics and cortisone in me. That only made me sicker. Now nutrient injections are helping, but I have a different problem. My insurance company will pay for poisons but not for nutrients.

Society's Choice

"This is what I think of our society's choice for us," a September canary said to me with sadness, "Going to see Kevorkian for dying? Fine! Go ahead. Going to a holistic doctor for living? Absolutely not."

Killing Machines and Breathing Devices

The enigma of why doctors forcefully declined non-drug therapies, of course, was not new. There was a long history of social contradiction. The American-born Hiram Maxim invented the machine gun, for which the English king knighted him. Sir Hiram also invented a steam apparatus for easing his recurrent episodes of bronchitis, for which the English doctors ridiculed him.

- When Sir Hiram tried to market his inhaler device, he was accused of profiteering—of, in his words, "prostituting my talents on quack nostrums."

- Before his death, Sir Hiram wrote: "From the foregoing it will be seen that it is very creditable thing to invent a killing machine, and nothing less than a disgrace to invent an apparatus to prevent human suffering."

A few integrative physicians also tried Sir Hiram's method —then designated hyperbaric oxygen therapy—for the September syndrome. The victims reported clinical benefits of the therapy. The problem again was that the insurers of the victims stubbornly refused to cover oxygen therapy.

The Killer Bubbles

An integrative physician observed considerable benefits of intravenous hydrogen peroxide therapy for victims of the September syndrome. He employed a very weak solution of hydrogen peroxide which was known to activate genes for important antioxidant enzymes. Beyond that, the low concentration of the liquid used seemed to normalize oxygen metabolism. Neither he nor his nurses who administered the infusions had observed any adverse effects.

The state licensing board investigated him. At one point, the head of the inquisitors angrily denounced him for using hydrogen peroxide therapy. "Don't you know hydrogen peroxide makes bubbles. How many people have you killed by those bubbles?" The accused physician replied meekly, " Sir, at that low concentration we have not seen any bubbles."

Pediatric Canaries

The City had a large number of pediatric canaries—children with poor constitution as well those with weakened immune system. By 2005, not surprisingly, many children in the City were also struck by the Malady.

There were two special considerations in the case of pediatric canaries: First, there was the frightening increase in the incidence of allergic, immune, and behavioral disorders. Second, there was the matter of their immune systems weakened by improper medical management. As for the first, consider the following quotes about the incidence of various disorders in pediatric canaries:

> As we approach the millennium almost half the population of the West demonstrates sensitization to one or more environmental allergens. In countries such as Britain or Australia, this translates to one in four children under the age of 14 years having asthma and one in five having eczema.
>
> *Nature* 1999;402:B2 (Supp)

> One in four school children in New York City carry an inhaler (to control asthma attack) to school.
>
> *New York Magazine*

One of every six children in America suffers from problems such as autism, aggression, dyslexia, and attention deficit hyperactivity disorder.

> In California, reported cases of autism rose 210 percent, from 3,864 to 11,995, between 1987 and 1998.
>
> In New York, the number of children with learning disabilities jumped 55 percent, from 132,000 to 204,000 between 1983 and 1996.
>
> *US News & World Report,* June 19, 2000

The second issue of the weakened immune system primarily concerned the disregard of pediatricians of the special nutritional requirements of those pediatric canaries and their disinterest in the matter of food and mold allergy. Many of those canaries lived on sugar and antibiotics. Their food reactions went unrecognized. Their mold and other types of inhalant allergies remained undiagnosed and untreated. Tonsils and adenoids were removed without performing tests for allergies. Ear tubes were inserted without regard to the underlying blockage of passages by allergic reactions. Wheezing was treated with steroids for short-term benefits but without regard to how those drugs suppressed their immune systems. The same was true of steroid creams used to control skin rashes and eczema. When sugar roller coasters triggered hyperactivity responses and attention deficit difficulties, Ritalin and other drugs were freely prescribed without regard to underlying nutritional factors.

The number of the pediatric canaries in the City had grown dramatically before the terror and toxicity of the Twin Towers arrived. After the disaster, pediatricians freely diagnosed what they called the Twin Tower syndrome and prescribed yet more drugs. They were neither trained nor interested in nutritional and environmental issues.

Tired Children, Teenagers in Pain

Within months of the September events, many children were unduly tired. Some appeared listless for periods of time. Parents observed the changes and took them to pediatricians who ran some tests and assured them that there was nothing wrong with the children. And so was the case with many teenagers. Other parents simply ignored—at great peril—the unexplained tiredness and listlessness of their children and teenagers with little, if any, understanding of the involved risks. Some blamed persistent tiredness on *children's blues*—a state not well recognized outside the City. Some blamed muscle pain and brain fog among teenagers on *hormone haze.* Amazingly, doctors expressed amusement at such notions about causation of fatigue, myalgia, and mentation difficulties, but did nothing to take the problem seriously.

Back in 2001, many parents had expressed concern about the barrage of bad news on TV. However, the media had stirred a national feeding frenzy for such news. There was no realistic chance of any parent protecting the children from it. After hlaf-hearted efforts, the parents simply gave up. The children received the blasts daily for months—from suicide bombers to exploding planes, from lethal bioterrorism to attacks with war poisons, from spraying poisons with planes used for treating crops to nuclear devices that could be carried in suitcases. The children and teenagers were not immune to such terror inflicted through TV screens.

> Treating the September canaries with antidepressants alone was intellectual bankruptcy, pure and simple—just it had been with the Gulf War canaries. We should have known.

Part 3

A definition of the basic molecular lesion in the syndrome.

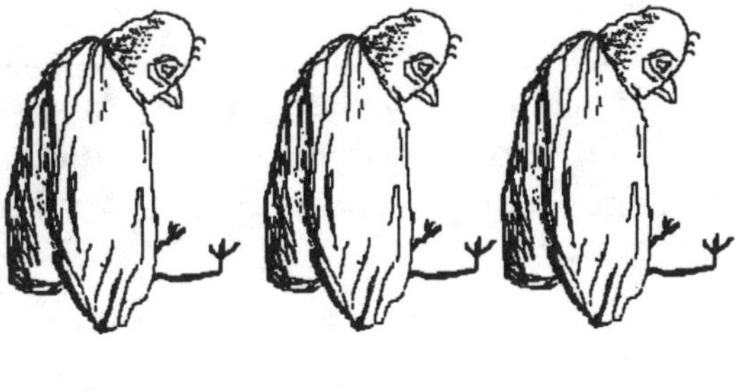

Windows on the World

A cell looks at the world around it through a million "eyes." The events of September Eleven affected *all* of those eyes in everyone. But the effects were long lasting for the constitutionally weak—they became the September canaries.

During the first twenty-six years of my study of medicine as a surgeon and a pathologist, questions about the causes of diseases fascinated me. Then I lost interest in those questions. During the last eighteen years, the single question of how can anyone ever remain healthy preoccupied me.

A cell is a living being of enormous complexity and intelligence. Free radicals are essentials to its life. Free radicals can also kill it. Enzymes build cells up—and tear them apart. Hormones program the behavior of cells for life—and for death. Antibodies guard cells from outside invaders—and turn against cells in autoimmune diseases.

The cell membrane reads its environment and alters its structure and functionalities to respond to changes in its surroundings. It changes its composition of lipids, proteins, and sugars to deal with alien molecules and microbes. It has channels, receptors, enzymes, and transporters.

There are an estimated 30,000 genes and 100,000 proteins in the human body. How do those genes create, shape, mold, and regulate those proteins? How do proteins regulate genes? How do those genes and proteins move in perfect harmony to produce a perfect baby?

The poet asks a question. The scientist spends a lifetime answering it, only to find that the poet has raised a much deeper question. How did September Eleven turn so many into human canaries? More importantly, how did the others in the City escape the terror and toxicity of the Twin Towers inferno?

Earlier, I wrote about the vast web and the enormous kaleidoscope of human biology. Every part of that web is connected to every other part. When something in that kaleidoscope changes in one way, everything in it changes in some way. Those were the two simple facts about human biology that the City doctors could not understand. The terror and toxicity of that September morning affected each fat molecule in the cell membrane, each sugar molecule in the soup of life within the cell, each protein molecule in the nucleus, each antioxidant system in the mitochondria, and, most significantly, each enzyme involved in the oxygen metabolism in the cell. *Each of those millions of eyes of the cell—windows on the world around the cell—was affected.*

How is it that everyone in the City was not turned into a September canary? That question preoccupied me.

Terror and Toxicity at the Cell Membrane

The cell membrane is an astounding paradox of fragility and resilience. The September Eleven morning abraded and lacerated the cell membranes of everyone in the City. The terror and toxicity of the Twin Towers turned into terror and toxicity at the cellular level. The resilent cell membranes of most people recovered from the massive trauma, but the fragile membranes of human canaries could not.

A cell membrane separates internal order from external disorder. It permits entry of what is needed inside (nutrients) and facilitates discharge of what is unneeded (waste). It keeps what is outside the cell from flooding the cell innards. It prevents what is inside the cells from hemorrhaging out. It converts physical changes in the fluid that bathes it (lymph) into chemical changes within. To do all that, cell membranes have many different types of communication molecules called receptors, which are especially vulnerable to environmental and metabolic poisons.

Cell membrane receptors are generally classified in the following five basic types: (1) those that detect and respond to mechanical factors (mechanoreceptors); (2) those that detect changes in temperature (cold and heat thermoreceptors); (3) those that are involved in pain sensation (nociceptors); (4) those that respond to chemicals (chemoreceptors); and (5) electromagnetic receptors, which are poorly understood and include light-sensitive receptors. I hold that the functions of *all* such receptors are regulated first and foremost by oxygen, though I recognize that evidence for that in some areas is lacking at this time.

The injured cell membranes hurt the September canaries in many ways. The two most serious consequences were:

1. The membranes of the canaries became leaky—what was inside the cells hemorrhaged out and what was outside flooded the cell innards; and
2. The membrane receptors, channels, and enzymes of membranes were structurally damaged and functionally impaired.

The above mechanisms explain the myriad clinical faces of the September canaries. Their muscles were weak and hurtful because magnesium within the muscle cells had hemorrhaged out. They felt 'dried out' because calcium in the blood had flooded their cell innards, switching on many destructive messenger systems of the cells. They suffered air hunger because their cellular oxygen enzymes could not survive the cumulative toxic overload. The female September canaries had irregular menses —many of them lost menstrual cycles completely—because their hormone receptors were blocked and damaged by chemicals that were structurally very similar to the natural hormones.

The basic question of what were the *initial* triggers for their cell channel operations (closing and opening) and receptor activation received little, if any, consideration from the City doctors. They had long abandoned their search for a specific entity—a disease—in the September canaries.

Terror and Toxicity at the Matrix

In the human body, matrix is the cement that holds the cells (bricks) together. The matrix of the September canaries was as vulnerable to environmental and metabolic poisons as their cell membranes and cell innards.

Matrix is much more than mere scaffold for the cells. *It both directs life inside the cells and is directed by them.* That is the basic theme of complmentarity in nature that I teach my canaries. Matrix and cell membranes form a continuum that directs intelligence to and from the cells. This continuum is directly and continuously exposed to oxidative stresses in the circulating blood and lymph. Thus, it is not surprising that the oxidative coals in the blood and lymph (microclots) will also sear the matrix and membranes. Indeed, the literature on patterns of injury to matrix and membranes is voluminous, and the thread that runs through all those events is oxidative injury that sets the stage for oxygen dysfunction.

When the September canaries bruised easily, injury to the matrix played an important role in that. When their wounds healed slower than those of others, the matrix was involved. When they experienced joint stiffness, the matrix in their ligaments and tendons had lost some of its elasticity. When their skin lost its vigor, the matrix of the skin had dried up. Indeed, many September canaries had told me that they had aged much in a period of just a few years. I knew their matrix was shriveling. The matrix plays key roles in all of those phenomena and in myriad others. Injury to matrix caused by environmental and metabolic oxidants and poisons was firmly established long before that fateful September morning. However, the City doctors were uninterested in the matrix.

Terror and Toxicity at the Nerve Cell

The September canaries often experienced palpitations and skipped heart beats. That was so because the membranes of their autonomic nervous systems could not maintain their potentials due to their toxic states. It had been known for decades that the autonomic system was especially susceptible to toxicity of PCBs, dioxin, and many other related synthetic chemicals. It had previously coined the term oxidative dysautonomia for a state in which cumulative oxidative injury interferes with the autonomic nervous system.

I knew from the early flashes of the TV images of the Twin Towers that symptom-complexes of oxidative dysautonomia will be among the most distressing for the canaries. So I was not surprised with the plethora of autonomic symptoms which included: temperature dysregulation (including severe sensitivity to cold temperature of Raynaud's phenomena; abnormal patterns of sweating; sudden episodes of nausea and profuse sweating; tachycardia, skipped beats and palpitations; episodic lightheadedness and/or dizziness; postural and orthostatic (neurally mediated) hypotension; dryness of mouth and eyes; urinary frequency and urgency; and fluid retention.) Symptoms of the dysfunction of the hypothalamus—an essential part of the autonomic nervous system situated in the central brain—included changes in appetite and sleep patterns. Another aspect of autonomic dysfunction that often went unrecognized and untreated was hypoglycemia followed by sugar roller coasters.

Brain fog and memory difficulties were caused by poisoning of other parts of the brain. The City doctors shrugged off those symptoms as mere stress response, albeit exaggerated.

Blood Turns Sour With Acids, as Milk Turns Sour With Lemon Juice

The white and the yellow of an egg harden when it is boiled. Milk turns sour and forms tiny curdles when a few drops of lemon juice are squeezed into it. It turns into yogurt when a culture of microbes is added to it. Those are three examples of how proteins in liquid form solidify when they are:

1. Heated (as in boiling of an egg);
2. Exposed to acids (acid in lemon juice turns milk sour); and
3. Acted upon by microbes (culture produces yogurt).

By similar mechanisms, the proteins in the circulating blood solidify into microscopic clots—microclots, in my lingo—when exposed to:

1. Excessive oxidative stress caused by lifestyle and biologic stresses;
2. Organic acids produced in excess during metabolic stresses; and
3. Enzymes of microbes (bacteria and yeast) and toxins produced by viruses and parasites.

The CUE and CUD of the Health/Dis-ease/Disease Continuum

Blood clots and unclots at all times. I recall many doctors raising their eyebrows when they first heard me say that. That did not surprise me since students in medical schools continue to be taught that blood in health is free of all microclots. There is, of course, no basis of such teaching.

I coined the term clotting-unclotting equilibrium (CUE) for a healthful state of the circulating blood when the unclotting process efficiently dissolves microclots formed in the blood so that such clots do not accumulate. The clotting-unclotting dysequilibrium (CUD) is my term for a "dis-ease" state of the circulating blood in which excessive microclot formation exceeds the body's unclotting capacity. The unclotting process cannot efficiently dissolve microclots formed in the blood, so such clots begin to accumulate.

> The simple fact of CUD cannot escape anyone with a serious interest in the microscopic study of the blood.

Oxidative coagulopathy is a term for formation of microscopic blood clots in the circulating blood. Blood clots and unclots at all times. In health, microscopic clots formed in the blood are readily dissolved so that such clots are seen infrequently in freshly prepared blood smears. When microscopic clotting is speeded up by any of the factors mentioned above, excessive microclots accumulate in the blood and are lodged in different parts of the body, choking the blood supply to that part and causing accelerated oxidative injury.

Table 1. Microscopic Features of Healthy Blood Smears	
1.	Clear plasma;
2.	Round red blood cells with smooth surface;
3.	White blood cells that move slowly like amoebae;
4.	Blood platelets seen singly or in small clusters;
5.	Minute fast-moving fat particles;
6.	Few cells with spiked, crinkled, or otherwise irregular outlines;
7.	Uncommon bacteria and other types of microbes;
8.	Rare zones of solidified (congealed) plasma, loose microclots, and compact microplaques.

Table 2. Microscopic Features of Oxidative Coagulopathy	
1.	Deformities of red and white blood cells;
2.	Zones of solidification (congealing) of plasma;
3.	Clumping and breakdown of blood platelets;
4.	Needle-like protein precipitates;
5.	Lumpy soft plasma clots;
6.	Microclots;
7.	Microplaques.

In the early 1990s, I described in detail the abnormalities in the blood of the Gulf War canaries as well other human canaries who suffered from chronic fatigue syndrome and fibromyalgia. I proposed that microclots and microplaques in the circulating blood clog blood capillaries—the tiny blood vessels in tissues that allow nutrients to enter the cell and waste substances to escape. Furthermore, stagnation of blood loaded with microclots and microplaques resulted in accumulation in the blood of a heavy load of oxidized and denatured fats, proteins, sugars, and other nutrients. That, in my view was the primary cause of persistent tiredness and unrelenting tissue pain of the September canaries.

I wrote stories for magazines for my canaries and articles for medical journals for doctors to elaborate my simple concepts about clotting and unclotting in the blood. Once I wrote:

> Muscle pain is oxygen deprivation. That is the simple fact of muscle pain in the September canaries. When a leg muscle cramps and wakes a person with intense pain, that is *local* oxygen deprivation in leg muscles. When an older September canary suffers from myalgia and hurts everywhere, that is *systemic* oxygen deprivation in muscles everywhere.

My writings had no impact on the main body of doctors. They simply were not interested in reading what they considered to be frivolous conjectures about any cause of injury to cells which they could not treat with drugs.

The Stagnant Lymph

Lymph is a thin, pale, colorless fluid that runs in microscopic tubules in the body called lymphatic channels. Lymphatic drainage is the term used for the process by which toxic acids and other toxins are ferried to the liver and kidneys (via the circulating blood) for removal from the body. Lymph is also rich in immune cells and antibodies, and so serves essential immune defense functions in the body.

Another interesting idea crossed my mind during my study of blood samples of my human canaries. It occurred to me that denatured liquid substances in the lymph form microclots and microplaques in the circulating lymph—just as those molecules form microclots and microplaques in the circulating blood. Such clots clog lymphatic channels, just as microclots and microplaques in the circulating blood block the flow in capillaries. I designated those processes as oxidative lymphopathy. I coined the term oxidative lymphopathy for a clinical state in which stagnant lymph in tissues causes generalized soreness, muscle pain, and joint stiffness.

So the examples of the white of an egg turning hard and milk turning sour with drops of lemon juice were as relevant to microclot formation in the lymphatic channels as clotting in the circulating blood. Excess acids denature fats, proteins, and sugar in the lymph as they do in the blood. Excess oxidants use up cellular antioxidants in the lymph just as they do in the blood. Milk turns into yogurt when a culture of microbes is added to it. Microbes in the lymph, unless killed quickly by immune cells, solidify the lymph in the same fashion. I kept on searching for simple analogies to explain my findings and notions of dysfunctional oxygen metabolism to my human canaries. Denatured (and oxidized) proteins, fats, and sugars solidify lymph, I explained to them, to form microclots when they are exposed to:

1. Excessive oxidative stress caused by lifestyle and biologic stresses;
2. Organic acids produced in excess during metabolic stresses; and
3. Enzymes of microbes (bacteria and yeast) and toxins produced by viruses and parasites.

Oxygen Directs Three Great Communication Systems of the Body

The human frame is a marvel of biology. How does a cell talk to its neighbors? How does a cell read its microenvironment and respond to it? How does it learn about the needs of individual cells in other parts of the body? How does it know what happens in parts of the body far removed from it? How do the body's fifty trillion cells cooperate with each other to maintain perfect health in a baby? And how do those trillions of cells work together to restore health after a life-threatening infection in which every cell of the body gets badly hurt? How do cells in one part of the body know others somewhere else are injured and face death? I see the hand of oxygen in all such happenings. Indeed, it seems certain to me that future research will reveal many more ways by which oxygen serves both as the main messenger and the principal player in all those events.

Oxygen does not earn its title of a great communicator in my opinion simply because it provides the living environment in which information can be sent and received. Oxygen is *the* information molecule. This is the main theme of this book. I present information about how oxygen governs communications in three major systems of the body:

1. The circulating blood;
2. The circulating lymph; and
3. The cell membranes.

Furthermore, I show how oxygen not only directs the flow of information in each of those communication systems but also serves as the principal medium of transfer of intelligence from one type of cell to another, from one type of tissue to another, and from one body organ to another.

> In two seemingly simple acts of clotting and unclotting blood, oxygen masterminds healthful aging.

The above may seem a wild statement to many. However, a few moments of reflection on what clotting and unclotting involves will make the meaning of my statement clear. The prevailing view that clotting in the circulating blood occurs only in phlebitis and a few other disorders is extremely limited. Furthermore, the view that clotting involves a small number of clotting factors is equally inadequate. In reality, clotting involves, directly or indirectly, *all* substances in the circulating blood (including enzymes, minerals, vitamins, proteins, fats, sugars, and organic acids). In addition, *all* cells in the circulating blood (red blood cells, white blood cells, blood platelets as well as cells lining the blood vessels) actively participate in the clotting process. Neither does the prevailing thought recognize that *all* substances in the plasma (the fluid part of the blood) as well as *all* types of blood cells are also directly or indirectly involved in the unclotting process.

Oxygen-Starved Tissues Hurt

I introduced the term dysfunctional oxygen metabolism for a cellular state when enzymes involved in oxygen metabolism are poisoned.

It became obvious to me that such blockage in the lymph channels will result in accumulation of toxic organic acids as well as other poisonous waste substances in the tissues. Furthermore, lymph blockage will impede the flow of blood in tissues and so interfere with the delivery of oxygen and nutrients to tissues. I had known for years that oxygen-starved tissues hurt.

Three Furies

Greek mythology fascinates me. The stories of the three Furies, it seemed to me, foretold the plight of the September canaries.

I call oxidosis, dysoxygenosis, and acidosis the three chemical furies in the plight of the September canaries—after the three evil Furies of Greek mythology. Like the Greek Furies, each September fury has a killing mission. Each is unrelenting in its pursuit. Each fury fans the flames of the other two furies. Thus, oxidosis, once begun, takes on a life of its own. Whether triggered by metabolic, microbial, or man-made oxidants, oxidosis not only fans its own flames, it awakens the other two fibro furies (dysoxygenosis and acidosis), and together all three unleash oxidants that turn rancid everything in their way, paralyzing all energy, digestive-absorptive, energetic, detox, and neurotransmitter enzymes of the body.

The Greek Furies were let loose by Greek gods infuriated by the misdeeds of mortals. The Greek gods were unpredictable and often became angry without reason. They were wont to abuse their godly powers and strike down mere mortals at whim. Zeus, the chief god, was the most volatile, often throwing his lightning rod for reasons known only to him.

The September furies, by contrast, are unleashed by the gods of greed. Unlike the Greek gods, the greed gods are consistent and predictable. They are the gods of the sugar, antibiotics, and pesticides industries. And of industrial pollutants, toxic metals, synthetic hormones, and radiation. Other gods of greed populate hospital committees, licensing and insurance boards, and medical journals. They *do* know what they do. They are utterly committed to profitability. How many children get hurt in their way is not their concern. How many adults are mauled is not their concern. How many elderly are numbed by their drugs is of no significance.

Oxidosis was the first fury. It was awakened by the buildup of oxidants in the body. This fury lacerated and mutilated every molecule, every cell, and every tissue in its way. It then awakened the other two furies: dysoxygenosis and acidosis. All three furies then fanned the fires of each other, cooking every molecule, every cell, every tissue they encountered.

On Banishing the September Furies

There is one big difference between the Furies of Greek gods and those of the greed gods. The mortals were defenseless against the Greek Furies. They knew not how to banish them. The September canaries, by contrast, are not so helpless. They can learn to banish the furies of the greed gods—with knowledge and defiance.

While the nature of the three September furies was simple to understand, the plans for banishing them were not to many. All of my September canaries eventually learned that they had to be kinder to themselves so their bodies can be kind to them. They needed strong nutritional support. They required vigorous detoxification measures. They benefited much from oxygen therapies. They had to learn to surrender to that larger *Presence* that permeated each of them at all times.

Furies are the Same, Only the Target Organs Change

There is one other great benefit of understanding the nature of the fibro furies and learning how to banish them. It turns out that the furies which unleash other diseases are the same as the fibro furies: oxidosis, dyxoxygenosis, and acidosis. Thus, what the fibro canaries learn to recover from fibromyalgia will also help them prevent other nutritional, immune, and degenerative disorders.

Sometimes I was carried away by my wandering thoughts, little aware of how my words created new fears in the heart of my September canaries. I was usually obsessed by that theme of three furies. The plight of my September canaries, I often mumbled to myself, cannot be understood without a full grasp of the three simple scientific facts of oxidosis, dysoxygenosis, and acidosis. Acidosis disturbed the delicate balance between acids and alkalies in the body. The changes in pH seriously interfered with the activities of enzymes involved in the digestive-absorptive, detox, neurotransmitter, and energy functions of the body. Acidosis was worsened as oxidosis and dysoxygenosis progressed. In turn, acidosis fed the fires of both oxidosis and dysoxygenosis. I insisted that no one could ever design any rational and scientifically sound plans for recovery from this syndrome without grounding all therapies on those facts.

Sometimes I told my September canaries my story of twin sisters, one of whom was a September canary. The twins were told to sprint one hundred yards on a beach on a day after a lightning storm when the beach air was crisp, clean, and free of air pollutants. Both were exhausted after the sprint. The healthy twin stopped to catch her breath and within minutes was ready to sprint again. That was not the case with the canary sister. She collapsed and stayed in bed for some days. There was evidently no deficiency of oxygen in the air by the sea, I explained. Nor in the lungs of the twin sisters. The problem with the canary sister was her poisoned oxygen enzymes. My September canaries understood well the lesson of the story. Some doctors who heard my story were not amused.

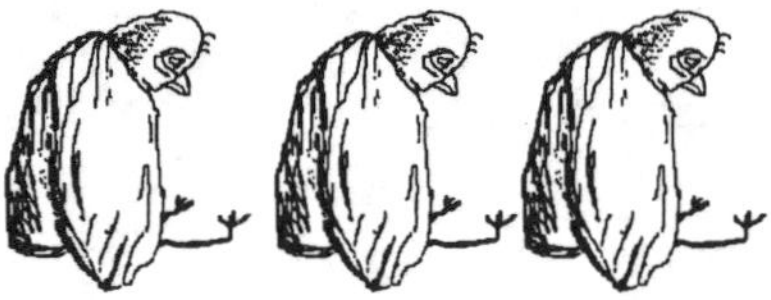

The Proof of Dysfunctional Oxygen Metabolism

A simple way to prove the presence of dysfunctional oxygen metabolism was to perform a test for 24-hour urinary organic acids. The September canaries also showed increased excretion of one or more acids—such as lactic, glyceric, pyruvic, and hydroxybutyric acids—in their 24-hour urine samples. Professional and advanced readers are referred to specific data obtained in my study of eighty-four persons with dysfunctional oxygen metabolism at www.jintmed.com.

The presence of oxygen dysfunction in the September canaries could also be demonstrated with examination of their blood samples with high-resolution and phase-contrast microscopy.

The Proof of Immune Dysfunction

The laboratory evidence for impaired immune status of the September canaries can be readily established by a variety of tests. In general, I have found the following two approaches especially useful.:

1. Demonstration of suboptimal levels of protective antibodies; and

2. Detection of abnormal and harmful antibodies.

Again, I refer professional and advanced readers to the Appendix for specific data comparing the protective antibody responses in a healthy subject to those in a September canary.

The Blood Cells Do Not Lie

I have had a passion for looking at cells and tissues with different types of microscopes for over four decades. From 1968 to 1996, I worked as a hospital pathologist with special interest in immune disorders. In 1986, I established an office practice and focused on issues of nutrition, environment, and stress. The environment, of course, included internal environment of the body as well as the external environment. Then I acquired a high-resolution microscope with phase-contrast optics for use in my office. That opened some windows to the world of cells and microbes that I had little inkling of.

During the late 1970s and early 1980s, I examined the blood samples of over 3,000 patients with immune disorders with high-resolution phase-contrast and darkfield microscopes. In that search I found a gold mine of information of immediate relevance to my patients—for a clearer understanding of the basic nature of their suffering as well as for defining the efficacy of various therapies I employed. In 1997, I described the following blood abnormalities in the persons with chronic immune disorders:

1. A large number of dead and dying red blood cells;
2. Damaged and dysfunctional immune cells;
3. Pine needle-like forms of curdled plasma;
4. Irregularly shaped clusters of aggregated blood platelets;
5. Minute curdles of blood plasma with trapped deformed blood corpuscles which are designated as microclots;
6. Irregular masses of compacted microclots with a layered appearance which are recognized as microplaques; and
7. Overgrowth of peculiar yeast-like microbes which multiplied

> rapidly when the amounts of oxygen in the blood samples (under the glass coverslips) fell. Several years earlier, I had called those peculiar forms of microbes primordial life forms.

I introduced the term oxidative coagulopathy for those changes and published my observations in several American and European medical journals. I also presented my findings in several national professional meetings. The mainstream doctors had no interests in such microscopic findings. That did not surprise me.

Oxygen and the September Canaries

For emphasis, I return here to the subject of oxygen dysfunction in the September canaries.

In the 1980s, I concluded from my microscopic studies that the *basic* molecular injury in human canaries was excessive oxidative stress—oxidosis, in scientific terminology.

In the 1990s, I began to focus on the problem of air hunger for the human canaries. I concluded from my microscopic studies that the *basic* molecular injury in human canaries was dysfunctional oxygen metabolism (dysoxygenosis) at the cellular level. I validated my microscopic conclusions by careful review of results of laboratory tests. I documented the fact that there was excretion of excessive amounts of toxic organic acids in the 24-hour samples of my human canaries.

Oxidosis, as indicated earlier, is too much oxidation. It is caused by the excess of oxidants. Theoretically, one should be able to correct it expediently by simply pouring into the body antioxidants to neutralize oxidants. That simply was not the case with my human canaries. That gave me my first clue that something much deeper was wrong with them. So, I conceived the basic notion of dysfunctional oxygen metabolism—dysoxygenosis (dys-oxy-ge-no-sis), in my lingo—when I observed that excessive oxidative injury cannot be simply controlled by the use of antioxidants.

Dysfunctional oxygen metabolism is caused by accelerated oxidative stress, which inactivates or impairs activity of enzymes of oxygen pathways. I call those enzymes oxyenzymes.

I discovered that dysfunctional oxygen metabolism was caused by events occurring either in the head or in the bowel. In the head, it was stress, anger, hostility, or confused demands for love. In the bowel, it was battering of the bowel ecosystem with unsuspected food intolerance, sugar overload, antibiotics, undiagnosed mold (yeast) allergy or overgrowth, and toxic synthetic chemicals. I insisted that all or any combination of those factors led, directly or indirectly, to dysfunctional oxygen metabolism.

Toxic organic acids, mycotoxins (toxins produced by fungal organisms), and other microbial poisons, I went on to explain, then spill from the bowel into the blood, and trigger the formation of microclots and microplaques. Next, those toxins poison oxyenzymes—yet another term I coined for enzymes involved in oxygen metabolism.

In that scenerio, the problems in the bowel and blood ecosystems next spread to the liver, which normally detoxifies toxins for the whole body. The liver, I claimed, failed to completely neutralize the toxin overload. That further worsened the degree of dysfunctional oxygen metabolism.

Proof of Toxicity in the September Canaries

Among the many frustrations of the September canaries was the claim of their doctors that all was well with them since all of their laboratory test results were within the normal limits. I knew better.

"What is the proof of your strange theory of dysfunctional oxygen metabolism?", a doctor once asked me. "Assuming what you imagine in the blood smears with your unique microscope is real," he taunted, "how do you jump to the conclusion that there is a problem in oxygen metabolism?"

That doctor had been told by cardiologists that they had found nothing wrong with the hearts of the September canaries. He had learned from pulmonologists that the same held for their lungs. Hematologists had found no proof of anemia in them. He was confident that if there were any *real* problems with persons considered to suffer from the September Eleven syndrome, they would have found them. Thus, the theory of dysfunctional oxygen metabolism to him was nothing but medical buffoonery.

He would find the proof if he ever bothered to measure toxic organic acids in the urine of those people, I told myself. Such exchanges were not uncommon, but were singularly of no benefit to the September canaries in their care. Their suffering was unremitting.

Three Main Symptoms of the September Canaries

More than other symptoms, what troubled the September canaries most was the complex of:

1. Persistent muscle pain (myalgia) with painful spots in soft tissues (trigger points);
2. Disabling fatigue; and
3. Brain fog (and related disorders of mood, memory and mentation).

Although victims of early and mild cases of the September Eleven syndrome suffered from one or two of the three main symptoms listed above, those with advanced stages of the disorder suffered from all three. Other symptoms included flu-like symptoms of malaise, aching joints, and abdominal bloating and cramps; bowel irregularities; non-restorative sleep; PMS symptoms and menstrual irregularities in women; cold sensitivity; and depression.

Simple Explanation of the Major Symptoms

To my mind, the mechanism by which the symptoms of the September syndrome were caused was straightforward. Disabling fatigue was caused by oxygen deprivation in all tissue. Persistent muscle pain was caused by oxygen deprivation in muscle tissue. Brain fog with problems of mood, memory, and mentation was caused by oxygen deprivation in brain cells. Air hunger was caused by oxygen deprivation within the cells. The last item required a special comment. Like other doctors, I had believed that the body learned about the lack of oxygen through special oxygen sensors in the brain as well as in the walls of large blood vessels in the chest and neck. My Gulf War and September canaries had forced me to look deeper into that issue. I could not explain the sense of air or oxygen hunger in my canaries merely on the basis of those oxygen sensors. Oxygen levels in the large vessels in those locations are within the normal range in victims of those syndromes. Thus, I had to look for some other mechanism. Then I came to believe that oxygen hunger was caused by abnormal oxygen metabolism within the cells.

Obsessed as I was with the notion of dysfunctional oxygen metabolism, I attributed all symptom-complexes of the September Eleven syndrome to dysfunctional oxygen metabolism— as I had those of the Gulf War syndrome. To me, that weakened the immune system, causing immune dysfunctions, such as sore throats, swollen neck glands, and painful tissues. Abdominal bloating, cramps, episodes of diarrhea and constipation, and problems of digestion and malabsorption were caused by oxygen dysfunction in the bowel. Cold sensitivity frequently noted by the victims was caused by poor blood circulation and oxygen dysfunction in the skin. I attributed sleep difficulties to oxygen dysfunction in the brain cells of the sleep center. Restless leg syndrome and leg cramps were attributed to such dysfunction in the muscle and nerve cells in the legs.

The problems of lightheadedness, dizziness, heart palpitations, and skipped heartbeats were blamed on oxygen dysfunction in the nerve cells and fibers that regulated blood pressure and controlled the heart rhythm. Dry skin, dry eyes, dry mouth, and dry vaginal tissues were produced when oxygen metabolism in those tissues became dysfunctional. Female September canaries commonly developed vaginal infections, while the male canaries reported prostate gland infections. That changed nothing for me. Dysfunctional oxygen metabolism in the immune cells renders them incapable of mounting war on the bugs, I had concluded. The canaries of both sexes often complained of poor sex drive. I blamed oxygen dysfunction in cells of the hormone glands for that.

Three Basics

I worked tirelessly to promote my idea that the fundamental energetic-molecular problem of the September canaries was dysfunctional oxygen metabolism. For every person who agreed to listen to me—and for others who curtly turned away—I had the same litany: (1) that all symptoms of the syndrome were caused by cellular oxygen deprivation; (2) that oxygen deprivation was caused by *dysfunctional* oxygen metabolism; and (3) that oxygen metabolism in the syndrome becomes abnormal due to excessive and cumulative oxidative stress caused by sugar overload, antibiotic abuse, undiagnosed allergies, synthetic chemicals, and anger.

Dysfunctional oxygen metabolism was neither merely a lack of oxygen in the air which the victim breathed nor in the blood that circulated in his body, I sometimes spoke with a preacher's fervor. Nor was it mere absence of oxygen in the cells. For me, it was a fundamental failure of enzymes involved in oxygen metabolism—oxyenzymes as I dubbed them.

The September Eleven syndrome, I repeated at the risk of annoying my listeners, had three Rs:

The syndrome was **R**eal;
The syndrome was **R**eversible; and
The syndrome could not be **R**eversed with drugs.

The September canaries were more vulnerable to unrecognized allergies, sugar overload, excessive antibiotics, and anger, and have been poisoned by synthetic chemicals. Those human canaries are telling us something important about the shape of things to come, I often murmured to myself. What injures their oxygen enzymes eventually will injure the oxygen enzymes of others, unless we find ways to protect the oxygen metabolism, I went on.

I seemed to tap into some inner spring of energy on those occasions. If you are a September canary, you *know* that the problem is real, I patiently explained to the victims of the syndrome. If your physicians doubt that, they cannot help you. Be kind to yourself and find another physician who understands this problem. The road to recovery from this syndrome is usually long and difficult. You need not make it much more difficult.

If you are a September canary, I would go on, please be kind to yourself and shun people who insist fibromyalgia is irreversible. The road to recovery from fibromyalgia is often long and difficult. You need not absorb the negativity of others.

If you are a September canary, I would conclude, please *know* that this syndrome cannot be reversed with any drugs. You *will* learn that sooner or later. No drug at present is known to cure the September Eleven syndrome. It seems highly unlikely that such a drug will be synthesized in the foreseeable future.

How can anyone be considered an expert on treating a malady that he can never effectively treat?, I asked in frustration. Why doesn't that question trouble the so-called experts who cannot help their September canaries?

Three Types of Poisons

I divided poisons that caused the September Eleven syndrome into three sets: (1) microbial poisons produced by overgrowth of various oxygen-hating microbes in the body; (2) man-made poisons that included pesticides and industrial pollutants; and (3) metabolic poisons generated during metabolism in small quantities under physiologic conditions and produced in large amounts when cellular oxygen metabolism became dysfunctional.

Of the three types of poisons damaging oxygen metabolism in my September canaries, I considered the metabolic toxins to be the least important in the initial stages, but the most dangerous in advanced stages of the syndrome. I explained that the reason for that was that all kinds of metabolic havoc were wreaked on the human tissues once oxygen metabolism becomes dysfunctional. The full significance of that statement became obvious—as far as I was concerned—when I found markedly increased amounts of toxic organic acids in the urine of my September canaries.

I defined metabolism as the sum total of all life processes that break down food substances for energy generation and prepare waste products to be gotten rid of. In my mind, in health the detox mechanisms of the body neutralized and cleared such poisons. In illness, those poisons were produced in such large quantities that the detox systems failed. Excess poisons accumulated in the body to cause oxidosis (too much oxidation [or breakdown]) which, in turn, led to dysoxygenosis (not enough oxygen), and acidosis (too much acidity). The state of illness that oxidosis, dysoxygenosis, and acidosis produced was what others called the September Eleven syndrome.

Microbial poisons were produced in large quantities by microbes which live in the body in health. Those microbes multiplied rapidly in the bowel and blood ecosystems with sugar overload, antibiotic abuse, pesticides, pollutants, and other toxins. All microbial oxidants cause oxidosis which, in turn, leads to dysoxygenosis and acidosis. Microbial poisons included those produced by: yeast species (mycotoxins); bacterial species (endotoxins and exotoxins); viruses (poisons produced by cells injured by viruses); and parasites (poisons produced by parasites as well as by cells and tissues damaged by parasites).

Man-made poisons, in my scheme of things, included the designer killer molecules (such as pesticides, fungicides, and herbicides), industrial pollutants, toxic metal compounds (such as dental mercury amalgams), and synthetic hormones. The toxic burden of chemicals had increased markedly during this century. The Department of Agriculture had reported more than nineteen million pounds of antibiotics were fed to cattle and chickens every year in the U.S. That was simply too heavy a burden of designer killer molecules for the September canaries to carry.

Three Molecular Mechanisms

In review, it became clear to me that there were three simple basic molecular mechanisms that inflicted molecular and cellular injury in the September Eleven syndrome:

Oxidosis (too much oxidation);
Dysoxygenosis (too little oxygen); and
Acidosis (too much acidity).

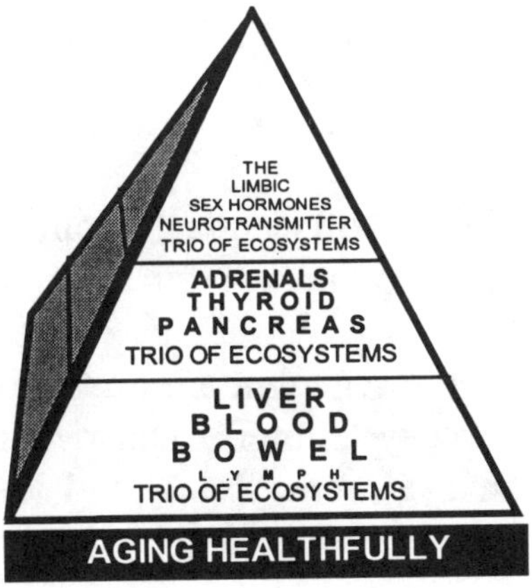

Three Levels of the Body Ecosystem

In 1998, I published a simple schema of three trios of the human organ ecosystems. That had evident relevance to my September canaries who showed—with what to me seemed ample clarity—how tissue injury spread from one body ecosystem to the other. I included the bowel, blood, and liver ecosystems and put the thyroid, adrenals, and pancreas ecosystems in the middle trio. My top trio of ecosystems comprised the limbic system, sex hormones, and neurotransmitters.

The Garden

The September canaries eventually recognized that their bodies were gardens. They learned that they needed to think and act like gardeners.

First,

they needed to work the soil regularly.

Second,

they could not banish every fungus (yeast), bug, or weed from their garden.

Third,

after they had seeded and tended the soil, they had to look up and *hope* for the sunshine and rain to bring out the flowers.

The soil in the divine garden of your body is the trio of the bowel, blood, and liver ecosystems. The canaries, first and foremost, must restore their damaged ecosystems, and then maintain them regularly.

Just as it is counterproductive to kill *all* living beings in the soil with pesticides and insecticides, one cannot do so in the soil of one's body with antibiotics, antiviral, antifungal, or antiparasitic drugs. The furies cannot be banished with synthetic drugs.

Just as a garden cannot show its celebration of colors without life-giving sunshine, the September canaries learned that they could not heal without the healing energy of hope and spirituality. Healing is an energy phenomenon. Hope is another word for healing.

The Killer Approach Did Not Work

A rose cannot blossom without bugs and slugs in the roots of the rose bush. The September canaries eventually recognized that they could not have clear minds and fair skins without a healthy bowel flora. Earlier on, most of them were told they had herpes, Epstein-Barr, cytomegalo, and other viruses. They were administered potent antiviral drugs. Others were told they suffered from Lyme disease, yeast, and parasites. Then they were prescribed powerful antibiotics, antiparasitic drugs, and antifungals. All such therapies had yielded limited short-term benefits but many long-term adverse effects.

1. Antiviral drugs destroyed their immune defenses long before they destroyed the last viral particle;
2. Antibiotics annihilated their bowel ecosystem long before they annihilated the last bacterium;
3. Antifungals badly damaged their liver ecosystems long before they badly damage the last fungal body;
4. Antiparasitic chemicals poisoned their cells long before they poisoned the last parasite;
5. Antimycoplasma antibiotics battered their bowel ecosystem long before they battered the last mycoplasma microbe.

Most antibiotics do not kill bacteria. They simply prevent microbial multiplication or reduce the rate of such growth. The killing of bacteria is left to the body's own hunter immune cells. The same is true for antivirals, antifungals, and antiparasitic drugs. No group of drugs listed above can banish oxidosis, dysoxygenosis, or acidosis. Indeed, all such drugs eventually facilitate the destructive roles of those three fibro furies.

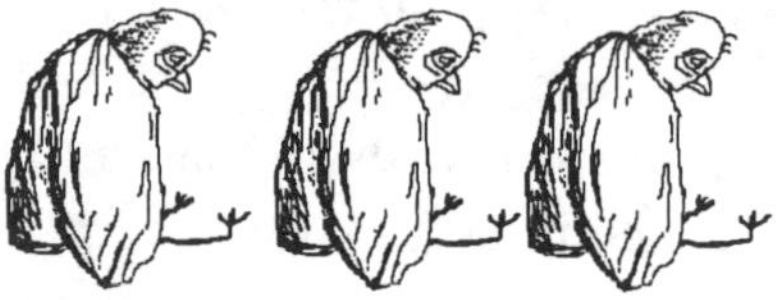

No shrine is holier than the human frame, for it houses the human spirit.

Caring for this shrine is a scared trust— sacred for the patient and sacred for the physician. It is this trust that sets medicine apart from other professions.

Physical disrobing of a patient for examination by his physician is symbolic of a deeper personal and emotional disrobing for the patient. And so it is that the simple act of a physician touching his patient establishes a unique bond between the two. This bond must not be breached by any expediency.

Molecular medicine is not an easy way out for the poorly informed physician...Nor is it an easy way for the patient. It asks for an ongoing pursuit of the knowledge of a patient's own biology.

The Cortical Monkey and Healing

Part 4

An explanation of how this syndrome could have been prevented, but why it was not.

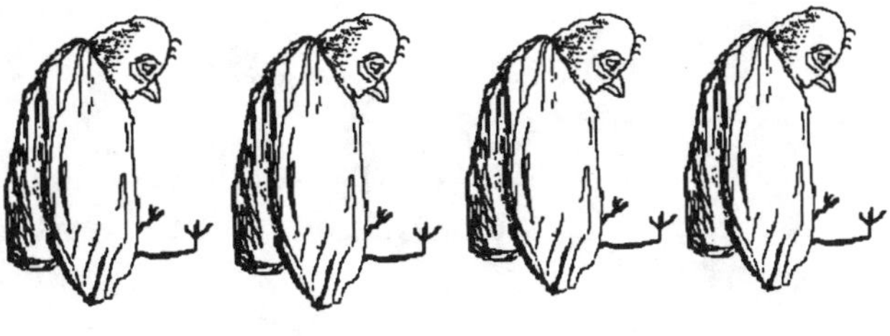

The Quack

It was midnight when I finished work with clinical charts and answered questions from my patients that the nurses were not able to answer. My long office hours usually did not create any unusual stress for me. I mostly saw patients with chronic immune disorders who had received little, if any, benefits from various drug regimens. Some patients made slow progress, but usually I was encouraged and sustained by positive follow-up reports. Even though the hour was late, I normally drove home satisfied with my work, sustained by a strong sense of having done some good for most of my patients. Generally, I tried not to think when I drove. I preferred a nonanalytical, meditative state of driving which I called the "limbic mode."

There were many victims of the September Eleven Sydrome in my practice. Most of them made slow and steady recovery. Some did not, and those patients preoccupied me. There were also times when some very ill persons in that group lost hope and became very depressed. Hope for them, I had discovered, was easy to create but hard to sustain. After listening to their stories, I sometimes returned home depleted in the mind and heavy in the heart.

After one such difficult day, as I prepared to leave the office, a nurse asked if I had a few minutes to talk to her. I glanced at my watch. It was some minutes past midnight.

"Is it about a patient?" I asked.

"No," she replied.

"Oh!" I wondered what it could be that she wanted to talk about so late. "Can we talk about it tomorrow?" I asked, looking at my watch.

"It will only take a few moments," she persisted.

"Okay," I yielded.

That nurse had joined our practice some months earlier. She often seemed uncomfortable with intramuscular and intravenous nutritional therapies. Initially, I attributed her uneasiness to the fact that she had been exposed to standard drug therapies and doubted that chronic disorders could be managed successfully without drugs or surgery. With passing weeks, I realized that perhaps there was more to her discomfort than the novelty of our approach. Perhaps it had something to do with our philosophy of medicine. Wrong time to discuss philosophy of medicine, I muttered under my breath.

"I have a question?" she began hesitatingly.

"I will answer if I can," I replied.

"The things you do..." she stopped in mid-sentence.

"What things?" I asked with a gentle smile, encouraging her.

"The things you do, are they legal?" She halted at the word *legal.*

"As far as I know." I tried to make my response as matter-of-fact as I could.

"I mean...these vitamin injections and drips." She was still tentative in her inquiry.

"As far as I know," I repeated.

"I mean...I know you are trying to get your patients off their drugs and that's what they seem to want. And I see that mostly you seem to be succeeding."

"Well, that's really the idea. Those patients need a lot of nutritional and immune support. Drugs simply do not work for them." I reassured her.

"But..." she again stopped without completing her sentence.

"But what?" I felt some irritation.

"But is it legal?" she reiterated her initial question.

"Are you suggesting that it is illegal to administer injectable nutrient therapies?" I looked puzzled.

"No! No!" she recoiled a little.

"Then what? What is it? What's bothering you?" I tried to hide my frustration

"I...I often wonder about these things, I mean I have never seen a physician use these treatment before. I simply wondered if they were legal why wouldn't other physicians use them as well?"

I forced a smile and told her that we would talk more about that subject later on. She was dissatisfied with the response, but thanked me.

I left the office with vague uneasiness. Minutes later, on Interstate Highway 80, I realized that what I sensed was more than uneasiness. It was bitterness, plain and simple. The office hours had been demanding that evening. I was weary even before the nurse raised the prospect that I was engaging in illegal activities. My thoughts drifted to a conversation I had with a colleague some months earlier. My colleague was very concerned with the direction of my professional work.

"Just be careful," he advised.

"Careful about what?" I asked in good humor.

"Be careful! That's all."

"What's this about?" I smiled.

"Don't get hurt, that's all." My smile seemed to irritate my colleague.

"I am not trying to get hurt," I protested.

"I am telling you to watch out. You can get hurt badly."

"You mean I'll ruin my reputation."

"Yes, that and..."

"And?" I peered into his eyes.

"There are yet other risks. You know that, don't you?"

"You mean my license can be in jeopardy?"

"Something like that."

"But what is it that I do that would jeopardize my license?" I protested.

"You know what!" my colleague responded testily.

"Know what? That my human canaries tell me that drugs do not help them. Injured antioxidant and immune defenses simply cannot be repaired with drugs that block some cell membrane receptor or channel. Others are simply not comfortable with the prospects of taking blocker drugs forever. That's why they see me in the first place. Is that a crime?" I asked with growing irritation.

"There is such a thing as prevailing standards of medical care," he continued.

"And the prevailing standards are drug standards! Is that it?"

"Yes! Yes! How else do you think anyone can evaluate your professional conduct?" he pressed on.

"Do you mean nutritional and herbal therapies and self-regulation are outside the prevailing standards?" I retorted.

"You don't understand something very basic," the colleague replied testily. "Let me put it this way. When someone gets a license to practice law in the state of Pennsylvania, he is required to practice Pennsylvania law. He is not permitted to practice New Jersey law. If he insists on doing so, he plays with fire. And if one day he loses his license, he alone is responsible for that. He shouldn't go blaming someone else for that."

"That's an interesting bit of logic," I said, hiding my sarcasm.

"It's not a matter of logic. It's a matter of law. The law says you have to be within the limits of the prevailing standards, and the prevailing standards are drug therapies," my colleague snapped.

"Drug therapies? And that's all," I said incredulously.

"Yes! Yes!"

"How does anyone practice preventive medicine with drugs?" I asked bitterly.

"I'm just telling you the risks you are taking. That's all," my colleague softened.

"I know you mean well. I know you are concerned about me. But I ask a serious question. How does anyone practice preventive medicine with drugs? How does anyone practice preventive medicine in New Jersey?"

My colleague looked at me for some moments, shook his head, and changed the subject.

The risk of losing one's license—and the only real means of making a living—is always alive with physicians who dare to defy the dogma of drug medicine and seek nondrug alternatives for their patients. Physicians who claim to practice preventive medicine are most vulnerable. How ironic! Practitioners of drug medicine regularly—and loudly—profess a strong interest in preventive medicine, yet they seldom miss an opportunity to insult those who actually practice it. And that is not where it stops. Physicians who practice preventive medicine using nutritional and environmental therapies are regularly investigated and frequently censored by their hospital and licensing boards. More than half of the members of the American College for Advancement in Medicine—in my view one of the two medical associations in the United States most committed to preventive medicine—are facing possible license revocation for their choice of nondrug therapies. (The second such association is the American Academy of Environmental Medicine.)

There were other flashbacks.

"Dad, why are you doing it?" the words of our son, Omar, then a medical student, came back to me. Sometime earlier, he had spoken to me about my clinical work. "You are on the faculty of a prestigious med school," he continued. "You were the chairman of a department in a major hospital for over twenty years. You have served as the president of the hospital medical staff. You have published so much. Why are you putting all that in jeopardy? Dad, why are you risking it all? Your reputation and everything else?"

I smiled at our son's questions but didn't give him any answer. As a medical student, I was also told by my professors that I must steer clear of quacks and charlatans in medicine, and that the surest way for a physician to destroy his reputation—my most precious asset—is to engage in dubious therapies. Like my son, as a medical student I learned that lesson well. I scrupulously shunned quacks.

A speeding truck rushing past me on the highway jolted me a little. I realized that what I was experiencing on the highway was not simple bitterness. There was a stone moving in my stomach, and every now and then it turned.

My unhappy thoughts wandered and turned to an annual meeting of American College Advancement in Medicine. I served as the program director. I invited a woman to the podium. Her physician-husband had been charged for professional misconduct for practicing nutritional medicine. A panel of experts for the prosecution had recommended that her husband's license be rescinded because he had administered unproven nutritional therapies. She spoke about the stark injustice of the case and how it was devastating their lives. She also made some comments about how they were thinking of surviving after the license was revoked.

Then she asked for help in paying the legal fees. She was a good speaker and delivered her message passionately, deeply moving the audience.

I had seen their beautiful three-year-old daughter some months earlier when I visited them to discuss the court case. During the visit, my host ran a video in which one of his accusers, a well-known nutritionist-hater, boasted about how he relished his hobby of putting nutritionists out of business. Suddenly at that moment, the little girl absent-mindedly walked in front of the TV set. "He wants to put me out of business," my physician-friend erupted with anger, and then suddenly broke down, "I look at my little girl and my heart breaks."

Some weeks later, I testified for that physician before a panel of experts appointed by an administrative court in the City. As expected, the court experts had never practiced nutritional medicine, and quite predictably knew nothing about the principles and practice of nutritional medicine. How do mainstream doctors maintain the facade of fairness, punish nutritionist-physicians and absolve themselves of guilt? I wondered. They ask other such doctors to serve as additional experts for the court. Such experts do not understand the principles and practice of nutritional medicine any more than those who sit on the investigative panels.

As I sat in the cavernous conference hall listening to the wife of my nutritionist-friend present her case, the details of the case flew through my mind. The government had no real case against her husband, but the prosecutors were determined to make him an example. It was evident that they were convinced he had perpetrated heinous crimes in denying his patients legitimate drug therapies. They wanted to teach him a lesson and they wanted to set an example for others guilty of practicing nutritional medicine they clearly equated with quackery. The day before I testified, Linus Pauling had graciously found time to testify for the defense. Pauling was the only living American to have received two unshared Nobel Prizes, one of which was for work in chemistry. I knew that one of the administrative law "judges" in the court was actually a retired high school chemistry teacher. Later I was stunned to learn that the court had declared Dr. Pauling's testimony inadmissable. Strange how things turn out for holistic physicians in courts of law! A retired high school chemistry teacher is an acceptable judge, but a chemistry Nobel laureate is not a suitable witness!

After that physician's wife finished, I went to the podium to introduce the next speaker. Out of the blue, words I had not prepared flew out of my mouth.

"What right does Tom have to put his innocent wife and their three-year-old daughter through such torture? What right does any physician have to put his family through such agony? What right does any physician have to deny his family of the only source of income he has: his license to practice medicine? What right does a physician have to bring disgrace to his family? What does his wife tell her family and friends? That her husband has been convicted of misconduct! What do his children tell their friends? That their Dad committed some horrible crimes for which his license was taken away! That they are destitute because the physician-provider of the family has lost his license and cannot provide for them anymore. And how do they explain why he lost his license? Would they understand that he was judged by a "judge" who, in reality, was a chemistry teacher and who knew nothing about the true nature of that physician's work? That he was convicted in a court of law because he gave his patients vitamins rather than drugs? Would anyone outside that court room ever really believe that such a thing can happen in the United States? People lose licenses because they do immoral things or they are incompetent. How would they convince anyone of his innocence?"

The audience, nutritionist-physicians and some family members, listened to me with silence that was loud with hurt.

"What right does Tom have to do this to his family?" I repeated. "What right does anyone else in this room have to do the same to his family? Why do we do what we do? Is it some form of self-flagellation? Self-aggrandizement? Delusions of being a savior? Or is it greed? Some get-rich-quick scheme? Charging big bucks for dripping nutrients into bodies to produce expensive urine, as some glib quackbuster put it? Why not go into surgery or radiology? Certainly there is a lot of easy money in those disciplines.

"Or could it be that it is stupidity? Sheer stupidity! Utter, unbelievable stupidity—losing it all for nothing."

"Prisoners of truth," I continued. "We are all prisoners of truth. Truth that sick people can get well without drugs! Truth that nutrients facilitate that process! Truth that drugs do not solve the underlying chronic problems of health! Truth that drugs work by blocking the very enzymes and mediators that we need for healing. Truth that as necessary as drugs are for acute life-threatening illness, the concept that drugs can promote health is fundamentally a flawed concept.

"Once we know this truth, we cannot back away from it. We see the dangers facing us. We see the risks our families face in this.

But we *are not* able to back away from it. Truth captures us. We are captives of the truth—prisoners of truth."

On the highway, my mind wandered from one traumatic event to another. I remembered a past president of the American Academy of Environmental Medicine who related to me an encounter with medical experts of the drug medicine in a court of law. "Do you have any idea what it does to you when you are called a quack in a full court?," he asked sadly, a residue of that hurt still alive in his voice. Then I recalled the words of another physician about his day before the state medical board. "I would rather face Gestapo colonels than those two-faced monsters." I nodded in sympathy. "A trifle melodramatic, isn't he," I told myself.

Why do physicians choose to become quacks? That question had never risen in my mind before. The first time I learned that someone—who knew nothing of my work—had used the word *quack* for me, it stung sharply. I looked it up in his dictionary. It defined a quack as one who, with little or no foundation, pretends to have skills or knowledge in a particular field...an untrained pretender to medical skill he does not possess, a fraudulent practitioner, an imposter, a charlatan. I recalled the dictionary definition of charlatan had amused, not angered, me—perhaps because by the time I looked up the definition I had recovered from the sharp bite of the word. Now my mind returned to that definition.

Little or no foundation—why are nutritionist-physicians considered quacks? Didn't they attend the same medical schools that drug doctors attended? Didn't they read the same texts? Didn't they take the same examinations? And pass them? What other foundation do they require to be considered physicians? A pretender! Pretender for what? That he is a physician, is that it? A fraudulent practitioner! Because he uses herbs? Or nutrients? Or teaches his patients methods for self-regulation?

An imposter! Who is he, a nutritionist, pretending to be a doctor? Oh yes! That charge does stick. There is a clear potential for deception here: Patients may visit him looking for toxic drugs and be tricked into accepting nontoxic nutrient therapies instead. Now that would be clearly wrong. The gullible public must be protected from such deception. Right! And the deceitful practitioner must be punished, his license revoked so that he cannot deprive anyone of his fundamental right to be drugged. An integrative physician must plead guilty to that charge—and be prepared to face the consequences.

What is it that nutritionists do that bothers the drug doctors so much? They learn the chemistry of enzymes and mediators and hormones, then use such knowledge in giving nutrient therapies. Why is that such a crime? What is it that clinical ecologists do that bothers the state licensing boards so much? They look for the cause of illness in environmental pollutants. What sort of crime is that? Who are they fighting anyway? Pro-pollution doctors?

Could it be that the real problem for the drug doctors is that nondrug therapies *do* work? Is that bad because it takes the drug business away?

What are you doing? A voice came from somewhere. At midnight, your own nurse investigates you. She quizzes you about what is legal and what is illegal in medicine. If you cannot convince your own nurse, what chances do you have with others? How can you possibly convince the investigators from the state licensing board? Your own son understands that. How can you explain yourself to other physicians?

You work till midnight. How many sick people can you care for? How many can you help? And how long do you think you can last like that anyway?

So you want to take a stab at Andy Warhol's 15 minutes of fame! Be known as *the* integrative medicine doc in the country. Is that the idea? *Tov sha berophem B' gehenem*—the best of physicians will go to hell—the words of the Talmud came from somewhere. You want to be remembered for your work? I mocked myself. To be known for insight? For speaking out against the dogma of drug medicine? For raising a voice against the tyranny of drug medicine?

Or is it a grand scheme for self-aggrandizement? The questions seemed to have no end to them. Is it a compulsion of an egomaniac? Some hidden, unmet inner need finding a socially acceptable excuse for spending long hours with the sick? The mask of a workaholic? What are you running away from anyway? Or could it be simple greed? This last thought stung.

Somewhere during that drive home I started questioning my work, something I did not remember ever doing before. I thought about quitting. Living a normal life like everyone else. The comfortable eight-to-five job of some HMO doctor perhaps. What morbid thoughts?, I scolded myself. All evenings free for those sitcom reruns on television, is that the substitute? And the news of muggings and murders. Some more time for eating out. Could that work for me? I grew more bitter with each passing mile.

The Black Bird

I entered my house bone-weary. I didn't recall ever feeling so depleted, so utterly disillusioned with work. My wife, as usual, was asleep in front of a turned-on TV set. I collapsed on the sofa next to her, low in spirit. The TV documentary was about a war which the country had fought in a far-off land over a decade earlier. In that war, the retreating armies of the enemy had put to torch enormous oil fields which burned for weeks, spewing monstrous clouds of toxic fumes. Enormous amounts of oil spills had run into the nearby gulf waters.

The documentary then showed a man wading knee-deep in thick slush on a beach. He carried a net on a long stick handle. In front of him and trying to escape from his net was a large black bird struggling with short, jerky leaps in the mud. The wings of the bird were smeared with thick, tenacious tar and mud. Each time the man neared the bird, the bird scrambled with jerky movements to move away. It evidently could not simply fly away. I watched this chase for some minutes. Gradually I realized what that chase was all about. The man with the net was a marine biologist from Chicago and the bird was one of the hundreds of thousands who got trapped in tar-slush when Saddam Hussein's soldiers let out enormous quantities of oil into the gulf water during the Gulf War. Some bird lover! I muttered. I didn't quite notice when the anguish of my thoughts about holistic medicine transformed itself into amusement at the plight of the biologist.

The scene on the TV screen changed, and I saw the man now holding the bird in his hands, trying to use a toothbrush to remove the gooey tar from its feathers. Gently and meticulously, the man worked on the back and the neck and the head of the bird. The scene changed again. This time the man held open the beak of the bird and tried to pour some pureed vegetables into its throat.

There is another fool, I laughed. How many Iraqi soldiers have been sacrificed? How many innocent civilians have been killed? How many Americans have lost their lives? How much ecologic damage has been inflicted on the region? How many hundreds of tons of toxic fumes went up with the smoke—only to settle down again over a much larger area? How many millions of gallons of oil flowed into the gulf? How many hundreds of thousands of those birds died in the tar? How many Iraqis and Americans will most assuredly develop an environmentally induced illness that will likely be designated something like the Gulf War syndrome? And this fool thinks he is saving the world by catching and cleaning a few birds! Funny stuff! And he is funny without trying, I mused.

Or could it be that it isn't about the sea birds at all? Did he come to save the birds or to save himself? Why did he fly all the way from Chicago to do just that?, I wondered. Wade in tar slush! Stumble around chasing some birds. What visceral compulsion drove him there? What inner demons is he appeasing—much like the ancients who would travel to far-flung hills to seek what they knew not? Or perhaps he is there to make a film—something to talk about. Something to write about. (Writers suffer from such need.) Who paid the bill? Must be some government grant money. No one would ever waste his personal money for such a trip. How much did it cost anyway to save the bird?

Or perhaps he doesn't know why he is doing what he is doing. Perhaps he is simply driven by his DNA sequences—programmed by some molecular arrangements that he knows nothing about, a captive of some visceral impulses he himself does not understand.

Then I saw the man from Chicago in me. You don't understand why he does what he does, neither do you understand what you do, the voice returned. You sit with individual patients, listening to them until midnight. What are you doing? How long are you going to kill yourself like that?, a physician-friend had asked me some years earlier. I had simply smiled back. Killing yourself for what? How many sick people can you care for? How many sick people can any physician care for? And in one lifetime? What are you trying to do? Save who? Your patients or yourself?, the voice sneered.

Why do men and women do what they do? Hillary climbed Mount Everest after many before him had perished on their way to the top. When asked why he did so, he is said to have replied, "Because it is there!" Is that all there is to it? Do we do things because they are simply there to be done?, I wondered.

Then it occurred to me that perhaps it was what the Holy Quran meant by *wajhah*—the divine determinism that exists beyond man's reach. Or perhaps it is what the ancient Hindus meant by *dharma*—allegiance to one's *core,* knowing the core being of a person, and doing what that core tells you to do. Perhaps it was the dharma of the man from Chicago to wade in the tar slush, chasing a sick bird. Perhaps I am like that marine biologist from the Windy City—staying up late with a few sick people doing what my dharma requires me to do. At the core, it does not matter how others look at one's work. Perhaps that is all there is to it—the *core being* of a person.

You keep doing what seems senseless even to yourself, I told myself. It matters not what your nurse thinks about it. Or what your peers in medicine think of it. Or what people serving on some state licensing boards think of it. Pity of others is something for them to dole out. There is no self-pity, dharma simply is to keep doing what comes natural to me.

Perhaps my son will one day discover that the professional reputation of a physician is not his most treasured thing, I thought aloud. It is a physician's *core being.* At that level, nothing but truth matters—the truth that a physician sees about the individual patient he cares for. The truth about what is safe and effective in the care of that individual patient. Unimpaired by concerns about his professional standing. Undaunted by the inquisitors from the state licensing boards.

I looked at my wife. She was in a deep sleep. I stood up, stretched my back, woke her, and together we went to the bed.

Part 5

An integrative plan for the prevention and reversal of September Eleven Syndrome.

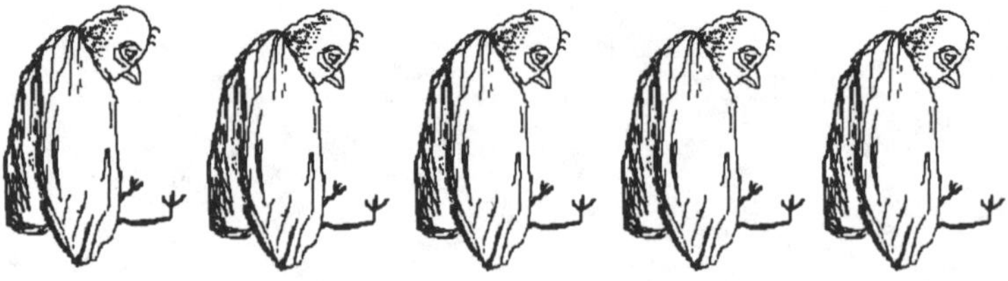

Seven Essentials of Recovery

In simple words, the September Eleven syndrome can be both prevented and treated by focus on the following seven essentials:

1. Restoration of the bowel health;
2. Cleasing the blood of toxic acids and metabolic toxins;
3. Detoxification of the liver of environmental toxins;
4. Reduction of the *cumulative* body burden of toxic metals and synthetic toxins;
5. Supporting the thyroid, adrenals, pancreas, and hormones with natural precursors of hormones;
6. Correction of *functional* nutritional deficiencies with nutrient therapies; and
7. Spiritual work (prayer and meditation) to *rid* oneself of anger and hostility, both of the kind that existed before September Eleven and that followed the onset of illness.

The above seven elements are essential for treating oxygen dysfunction and for restoring the cellular oxygen metabolism of the September canaries.

I often learn from the September canaries of their search for the "missing link." Many of them have the sense that they would recover if only some practitioner could supply that link—some nutrient, some hormone, some enzyme. Years of work with human canaries have convinced me that there is no such link. One needs to think and work like a gardener—always looking for ways to nourish the body, sustain it, and protect it from toxic substances.

Three Core Concepts

My guidelines for prevention and reversal of the September Eleven syndrome are based on my three core concepts of the cause and treatment of the syndrome:

1. Oxidosis (too much oxidation), acidosis (too much acidity), and dysoxygenosis (oxygen dysfunction) are the three primary molecular lesions of the syndrome;
2. The integrity of the bowel, blood, and liver ecosystems is essential to health—and disruption of those ecosystems leads to and perpetuates the September Eleven syndrome; and
3. Validation of all management plans must be done with long-term true-to-life clinical outcome studies.

Among the molecular lesions, I emphasize oxygen dysfunction because, in my experience, the progress in the other two (oxidosis and acidosis) simply cannot be maintained for long unless the oxygen metabolism can be fully restored. I support my dysoxygenosis theory with a large number of clinical and experimental observations summarized in *Oxygen and Aging*.

Among the ecosystems of the body, I emphasize the state of bowel ecology because, in my experience, the progress in the other two (the blood and liver ecosystems) simply cannot be maintained for long unless the bowel issues are fully addressed. Below, I include a simple schema that establishes my clinical priorities in my ecological thinking.

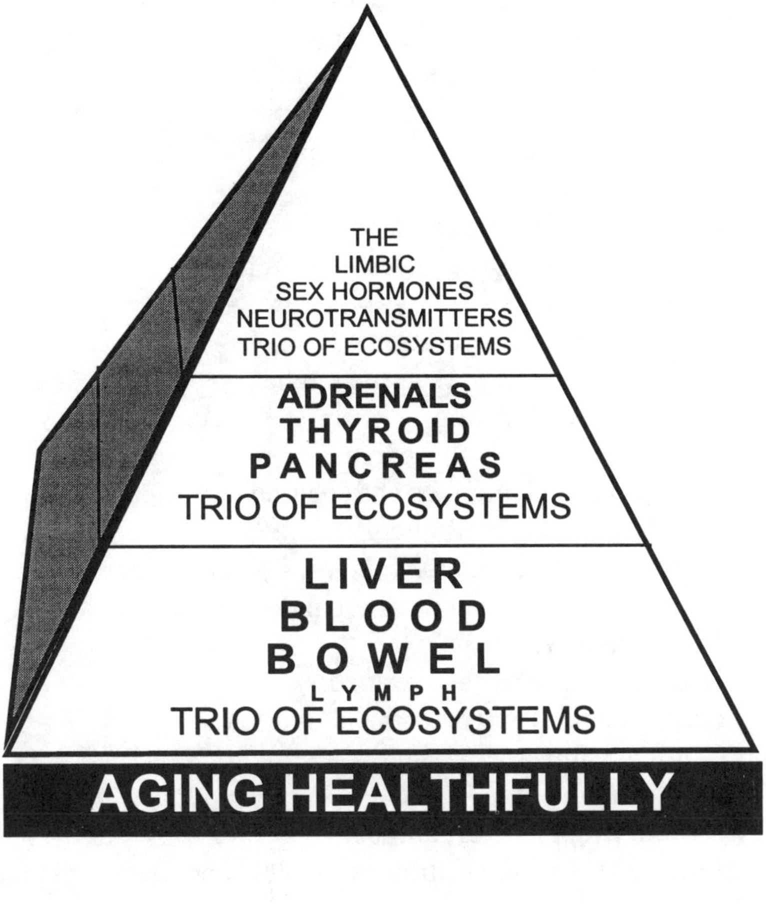
THE
LIMBIC
SEX HORMONES
NEUROTRANSMITTERS
TRIO OF ECOSYSTEMS
ADRENALS
THYROID
PANCREAS
TRIO OF ECOSYSTEMS
LIVER
BLOOD
BOWEL
LYMPH
TRIO OF ECOSYSTEMS
AGING HEALTHFULLY

Nineteen Elements of the Program

My clinical application of the three core concepts of the September Eleven syndrome presented in the preceding pages includes the following elements:

1. Resolving anger;
2. Healing love;
3. Understanding spiritual needs;
4. Stretching and gentle physical exercise;
5. Restoring sleep;
6. Assuring optimal hydration;
7. Avoiding poor choices in the kitchen;
8. Relieving constipation;
9. Avoiding sugar-insulin-adrenaline roller coasters;
10. Managing food allergies and incompatibilities;
11. Treating mold (yeast) allergy;
12. Reducing environmental (chemical) sensitivities;
13. Correcting functional nutritional deficiencies;
14. Balancing hormones;
15. Reducing toxic metal overload;
16. Diminishing synthetic cemical overload
17. Cleansing the bowel;
18. Cleansing the blood;
19. Detoxifying the liver; and
20. Intramuscular and intravenous nutrient and oxygenative therapies.

In the following pages, I include brief comments about each of the above elements. The common goal of work in all of the above, as indicated earlier, is to restore oxygen metabolism by: (1) restoring the various body ecosystems; (2) providing optimal nutrient support; and (3) reducing the cumulative body burden of toxins; and (4) spiritual dissolution of anger.

1. Resolving Anger

My human canaries have taught me two lessons about anger. First, angry persons do not heal well. Second, the answer to the problem of anger is spirituality, not psychology.

Psychologists and psychiatrists recognize anger as the root of many disorders. That has also been my observation. They think the solution to the problem of anger is in verbal unleashing of the hidden rage. They prescribe therapies for empowerment and control. I have not seen those approaches work well in the long run.

Neither the chemistry nor the energetics of anger have been worked out. Yet, based on my work with many angry canaries, I concluded that *anger is a powerful oxidizer*. And I am certain future research will clearly establish that. On a basic level, acute anger causes muscles to tighten up, and that produces local excess of free radicals, lactic acid, and other toxic organic acids (such as pyruvic, glyceric, and 2-hydroxybutyric acids). For the human canaries, chronic anger is worse and causes chronically tightened muscles, producing chronic oxidosis and acidosis, both of which lead to local as well as systemic oxidosis and dysfunctional oxygen metabolism.

Anger is a child of the thinking mind—the cortical monkey, in autoregulation language. That monkey cannot be banished with mere words. Indeed, he thrives on clever schemes and convoluted theories. The mind forever recycles past misery and, when that is not enough, precycles feared future misery.

Healing is not an intellectual function. No clever mind can order healing in injured tissues. The cortical monkey decorates doubt. It embellishes fear. Clever thinking is of little value in coaxing rebellious muscles to abstain from excessive contraction. Human canaries know that the pain of muscle spasm in the back or neck cannot be relieved by mere talking. Nor does the deep anguish of depression abate with so-called positive thinking. What is needed is *true* spiritual surrender.

Myalgia (pain in muscles) in the September Eleven syndrome is caused by a lack of oxygen in the muscle cells and by increased sensitivity of those cells to *local* oxidosis and acidosis. I have put local in italics because this matter is rarely appreciated by most doctors. More than one pulmonologist has criticized my use of nasal oxygen to treat severe pain of human canaries. Their reason for rejecting my therapy was that their blood oxygen studies showed what they consider a normal level of blood oxygenation. Similarly, some cardiologists could not understand why I prescribed oxygen for persons claiming to be victims of the Twin Tower horrors. The fact that oxygen therapy had clearly helped those canaries—as attested by the canaries themselves—was dismissed by those doctors as a placebo effect. That amused me.

The May 24, 2001, issue of *The New England Journal of Medicine* carried an interesting report.The authors surveyed dozens of articles which explored the issue of the efficacy of the placebo effect in diverse clinical conditions. From their extensive review, they concluded that the placebo has no real effects at all. That created an interesting scenerio for me: the placebo effect works for nutrient therapies—as claimed by pulmonologists and cardiologists—but not for drug regimens as pronounced by the *Journal*.

2. Healing Love

My human canaries have taught me another important lesson: *Love, like water, flows only one way*. It may be offered, but cannot be demanded.

Sending love sustains one,
demanding love depletes one.

Demands for love are demeaning. Facilitating the healing process in others by offering love, on the other hand, has a powerful healing influence for the victims. The ancients recognized that and counseled the sick to try to find ways to serve others. In my native Urdu language, the word for that is *saadhaqa (saa-dhaa-kaa)*. To my knowledge, all religions and all earlier cultures emphasize that. Even the sacrificial rituals of the ancients, in my view, were in recognition of the same phenomena. (Though, it seems to me, that the *spirits* they thought were mad and needed to be appeased by their sacrifices were really not mad.)

In *What Do Lions Know About Stress?*, I suggest several ways to reach out and serve others, including helping an elderly person in ordinary chores, befriending a sick child, or being kind to an animal. This path to healing is especially needed by those who have been chronically sick. To paraphrase John Ruskin,

> The true reward for one's service to others is not what one receives for it, but what one becomes by it.

The core aspect of this path to resolving anger for healthful aging is the matter of simply being present with the sick or the needy. Telling a severely depressed person to cheer up is a cruel joke. The same holds for common utterly frivolous platitudes used by people when speaking with the sick or grieved.

> A true gift of service is the gift of presence, and the essence of that presence is listening to what goes unspoken.

Another practical aspect of compassion through silence is that it is usually difficult for the visitor to divine what troubles those who are suffering and who need comforting most. What such persons need most is to be with someone. Of course, when that person is ready to say anything, she knows she is free to speak up. Thus, the easiest thing for the visitor is to simply *be.*

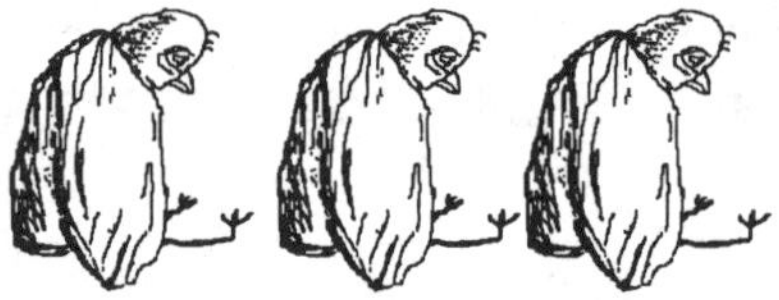

We can only as much divinity as exists within us.

3. Understanding Spiritual Needs

The third important lesson taught me by my canaries is this: Spirituality is a language without words. As long as one continues to struggle to define what spirituality is, one is out of it. That is the fundamental limit of humankind.

The wisdom of the ancient notion of mind-body-spirit trio is this: Whatever can be sensed with physical senses or perceived by the mind cannot be spiritual. For the spiritual to be discrete from the body and the mind, it must be beyond the reach of either. One cannot reach the spiritual either by seeing, smelling or hearing clearly—nor by superior thinking. Indeed, if that were true, there would be no need for the trio; the mind-body duo would have sufficed. How does one go about searching for the spiritual? One doesn't!

The spiritual has something to do with surrendering in silence to the larger *Presence* that permeates each of us. Why is silence essential? Because sights, smells and other sensory perceptions are aspects of the physical body—and language is the mind's turf. None of that constitutes the core of the spiritual. Clever thinking, after all, is just that: thinking. And thinking, by definition, is not spiritual. A thinking mind cannot *know* the spiritual.

For many September canaries, the mind becomes a tyrant—the relentless chatter of that monkey becomes insufferable. What that monkey cannot cope with is the silent energy of the spiritual. Specifically, I make two suggestions that I have found to be clinically useful: meditation with the silence of a candle flame in winter, and with the silence of stone during summer. In essence, we can only hope that through a candle flame or a stone we will enter that domain and experience some of our essential link with the larger Presence. These two simple approaches are usually far more rewarding—and revealing—than any elaborate ritual created by shrewd schemes.

Happiness is an illusion. That is one reason why no two people ever agree on what constitutes happiness. No matter which way one chooses to define happiness, it is an empty notion—now you have it, now you don't.

> Few things make people more unhappy than the search for happiness.

The best reason for practicing gratitude I know is that it makes getting out of the bed in the morning less demanding. For others, it makes the morning hours a profoundly spiritual time.

Gratitude, of course, cannot be gained with clever rituals or by traveling to exotic places either. It can be practiced anywhere, at any time. It requires neither any outside support nor any special inner capacity. I have seen patients who lived with profound gratitude even when they suffered progressive paralysis of body muscles by disorders such as multiple sclerosis and Lou Gehrig's disease (amyotrophic lateral sclerosis). I know of many young people who are incarcerated in their homes with incapacitating fibromyalgia, chronic fatigue state, and other chronic disorders. And yet, they are grateful for simply being alive. I know many chronically ill patients and angry persons for whom the word gratitude is a cruel joke. Then there are those who live in rage but do not quite understand why they are consumed by it. Both groups need a lot of work with the wordless language of spiritual awareness. Those who persist *always* succeed. Then they learn what is known to *all* who choose that path. Gratitude is a river that flows endlessly, neither revealing its true origin nor its destiny.

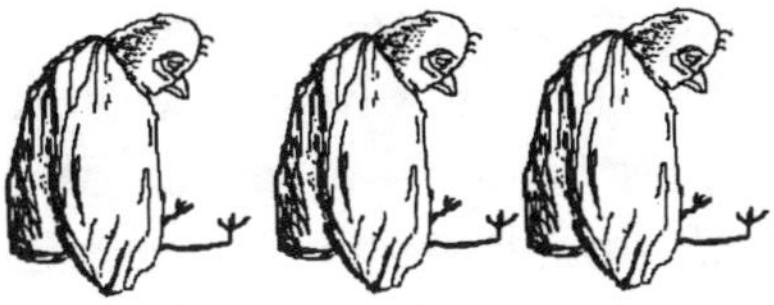

Silence can bring suffering or serenity depending on what we keep—and from whom.

4. Stretching and Gentle Physical Exercise

Limbic exercise is my term for slow, sustained, noncompetitive and non-goal-oriented exercise. This is an essential issue for the human canaries. Any exercise that leaves them tired ten minutes after they finish or the next day is actually harmful. The fundamental molecular lesion—I repeat often in this book for emphasis—is dysfunctional oxygen metabolism. Most commonly used exercises for physical fitness lead to a rapid buildup of acidity in the tissues of those canaries which, in turn, fans the smoldering coals of oxygen dysfunction. Thus, the September canaries need to be circumspect about physical activity. On the other hand, the September canaries have sluggish blood and stagnant lymph. Both factors cause stiffness of muscles and soreness in tissues. The best approach to those knotty problems is gentle but frequent stretching that covers *all* parts of the body. And that is what I emphasize to my canaries most for physical fitness.

Stretching followed by gentle limbic exercise done every morning, in my view, is essential for the September canaries. The core philosophy of such exercise is to integrate physical activity with a deep spiritual awareness.

How does an African tribal messenger run on his wilderness trail? What state of energy is he in? How does an American executive run on his sidewalk? What does his cluttered head demand from his tired and hurt tissues? How do hurt tissues rebel? Can physical exercise provide a deeply personal, treasured retreat from the relentless chatter of the thinking mind? There are important clues for the September canaries in those questions.

Roosters flutter their wings to announce their morning. Canaries flap their feathers before they fly off their nests. Dogs stretch before they take their first steps. So do cats. We humans wake up to our coffee and begin to recycle the misery of our yesterdays and map out the feared future suffering of our tomorrows. Those are some of my other thoughts on the subject.

The core notion of limbic exercise is well expressed in the following words of Lao tzu in Tao te Ching:

> ...a state of body awareness in which the right stroke or the right movement happens by itself, effortlessly, without any interference of the conscious will....The game plays the game; the poem writes the poem; we can't tell the dancer from the dance....the doer has wholeheartedly vanished into the deed....It happens when we trust the intelligence of the universe in the same way that an athlete or a dancer trusts the superior intelligence of the body.
>
> (Translated by Steven Mitchell)

5. Restoring Sleep

As is the day, so is the night. That, in simple words, is the *full* story of sleep disorders, I explain to my canaries.

I know the above statements will draw some chuckles from sleep specialists, who will consider them amusingly simple-minded. I have good reasons to support my view. There is an ever-growing list of sleep disorders in the United States today. Consider the following quote from *Science News*:

> Much controversy surrounds the definition of sleep disorders....Many sleep specialists criticize DSM (*Diagnostic and Statistical Manual of Mental Disorders*) for ignoring physical ailments linked to sleep problems, and some prefer an alternative classification that lists nearly 70 sleep disorders.

Nearly 70 sleep disorders! But how relevant is such a classification to those who do not sleep restfully? How common is sleep difficulty in the United States? Consider the following quote from *The New England Journal of Medicine* (1993:328:1230):

> The estimated prevalence of sleep-disordered breathing, defined as an apnea-hypopnea score of 5 or higher, was 9 percent for women and 24 percent for men....Undiagnosed sleep-disordered breathing is associated with daytime hypersomnolence.

Twenty-four percent of young men! The authors of the article studied a random sample of 602 young corporate employees. The important question here is: Why does one of every four young men in corporate America not sleep well? Or, to be more blunt, what is it that corporate America does to its young men to create such frequency of sleep disorders? On a larger scale, what keeps people everywhere restless during sleep? Why is sleep not deep and sound for so many people? Why do so many people wake up tired and stale?

When one sleeps, one is not dead. The state of sleep must be accepted as a continuation of the conscious state. How do adverse food reactions interrupt sleep? How do bowel problems interfere with sound sleep? What are the effects of muscle and joint pain on the depth of sleep? How does chronic anger change the quality of sleep? How do lifestyle and work stressors influence the sleep patterns? Those are the important questions. I rarely see sleep specialists make any *real* efforts to address those issues. Consider another quote from the *Journal* article cited above:

> Evaluation by current standards includes full-night polysomnography, at a cost per procedure of approximately $1,100. Sleep-disordered breathing can usually be eliminated by the nightly use of a nasal device that delivers continuous positive pressure to the upper airway. Since patients must continue to receive this therapy throughout their lives, it is often viewed as a hardship.

The *Journal* did not address any of the real issues concerning the causes of poor sleep I raise above. What they seem to advocate is that the use of sleep machines should not be viewed as a hardship. How can anyone sleep with his face covered with a mask and not find that a nuisance? Or have a tube stuck up his nose for several hours and not consider that a hardship? Years before the events of September Eleven, 2001, the *Journal* was very clear about the solution to the problem of poor sleep.

There is a growing tendency among sleep specialists to attribute various patterns of ill health to sleep disorders. That certainly happened in the September Eleven syndrome. The sleep "disorders" in the September canaries were caused by the same mechanisms that caused their other symptoms. As a matter of fact, my colleagues and I have managed nearly 5,000 human canaries—successfully, in most cases—with natural restorative therapies. When their damaged bowel, blood, and liver ecosystems are restored, they get better and their sleep disorders disappear. Most of the September canaries do need specific measures to restore sleep—such as meditation, music therapies, and natural sleep-enhancing substances, including melatonin, valerian, SAMe, tryptophan, passionflower, inositol, niacinamide, and St. John's wort. In certain cases of advanced sleep apnea—such as those associated with severe obesity, extreme cases of restless leg syndrome, and intense anxiety—the temporary use of a sleep machine may become necessary. But similarly, in chronic illness associated with chronic sleep deprivation, use of prescription sleeping pills is often advisable.

Following are three suggested plans for chronic sleep disorders. Even when prescription sleeping pills are necessary, I recommend one of the following natural plans to reduce the use of drugs.

Suggested Sleep Plans

PLAN A

1. For 60 minutes before bedtime, very low-volume music and meditation only. Specifically, no reading, talk radio or TV. Only very low-volume instrumental music or water-wave sound tapes.
2. Items to be taken in any combination at bedtime for three to four days a week:

   Magnesium, 500 to 1000 mg
   Melatonin, up to 12 mg
   Passionflower drops (up to 20 drops per time), may take it two to three times during the night if sleep is interrupted
   5 HT, 50 to 150 mg
   Hibiscus tea

PLAN B

1. For 60 minutes before bedtime, very low-volume music and meditation only. Specifically, no reading, talk radio or TV. Only very low-volume instrumental music or water-wave sound tapes.
2. Items to be taken in any combination at bedtime for three to four days a week:

   St. John's wort, up to 900 mg
   SAMe, 200 to 600 mg
   IP-6, 2 tablets
   Magnesium, 500 to 1000 mg
   Chamomile tea

PLAN C

Inositol, 250 mg
Niacinamide, 50 to 75 mg
Diphenhydramine, 25 to 75 mg (generally available)
(Benadryl is the trade name, but it does not work well for some)

6. Assuring Optimal Hydration

Next to spiritual silence, my first and best prescription for oxidosis is water. The same is true for acidosis. Next to spiritual silence, my first and best prescription for dysoxygenosis is also water.

Chronic dehydration was nearly always present in my September canaries. Physicians generally diagnose dehydration by testing for dryness of tongue and skin. That, of course, works only in advanced stages of dehydration in acutely ill persons and is wholly inadequate for determining whether or not a chronically ill person is optimally hydrated. That statement can be easily validated by doing the following test:

> An experienced clinician first helps the person to achieve optimal hydration for two weeks. That person is then asked to describe his overall sense of well-being. The next step in the test is to ask that person to limit his water intake to the pretest level for two weeks and again describe the general state of well-being or lack of it.

I conducted the above test for many human canaries. Nearly all of them reported some benefits of optimal hydration with the above simple test.

I prescribe water *therapy* for every September canary. I discuss water therapy and the state of hydration during almost *every* visit with each patient. The most basic reason for water therapy is the dilution effect of drinking additional water. It simply carries the excess oxidizing substances as well as toxic acids into the urine. Water is equally important to the integrity of all three major ecosystems of the body. In the bowel, water is the *single* most important laxative. In the blood, water is the single most important *functional* antioxidant. Without water none of the antioxidant enzyme systems of the blood can function well. The same is true for the liver ecosystem.

One of the fundamental differences between the cells in the body of a seven-year-old and a 70-year-old is that the cells in the older person are dehydrated, dried out, and shrunken. *All* cells need to be optimally hydrated to carry out their functions. None of the cell membrane channels, receptors, enzymes, and organelles can function well without optimal hydration. For example, neurotransmitters in the brain literally are like buds that do not bloom well without water.

My September canaries frequently complain that they need to drink large quantities of fluids to take their prescribed nutrients and herbs. I tell them that is good news. Nutrient protocols force them to increase their water intake. So much the better! The simplest and most effective practical measure for correcting acidosis, oxidosis, and dysoxygenosis is to dilute the toxins and eliminate them with increased fluid intake. Parenthetically, one of the fundamental changes of the general aging process is cellular aging. Aged cells are shrunken and dehydrated. The September Eleven syndrome is clearly a state of accelerated molecular and cellular aging. A state of overhydration is not only desirable, but necessary.

One-third of kidney diseases in the United States are caused by anti-inflammatory painkillers, many antibiotics, and contrast media used for scans. When the use of such drugs or contrast media becomes necessary for the September canaries, the simplest and most effective safeguard against kidney damage is optimal hydration.

"What is an optimal state of hydration?," many canaries ask me. Depending on the size of the patient, I recommend from three to five quarts of water a day. I advise them that organic vegetable juices and prescribed herbal teas may be considered part of that volume of water. Coffee, cocoa, caffeinated sodas, and black tea and alcohol are not to be included. In reality, under many circumstances such beverages are dehydrating.

I drink fifty to fifty-five ounces of water with nutrient supplements in the morning. This amount of fluid includes my breakfast, in which I put one and one-half heaping tablespoons of soy or rice protein powder in eight ounces of organic vegetable juice and then add another eight ounces of water to it. Such fluid intake assures me a state of overhydration and obviates any need for coffee or tea. A few trips to the bathroom are a small price to pay for the overall benefits of such a state of overhydration during the morning hours. How can I take so much fluid on an empty stomach?, some readers may ask. I take the stated quantity of water in portions of eight to ten ounces during twenty to thirty minutes of my limbic exercise. Readers may wish to add a piece of fruit to their protein drink for additional support or add small amounts of fruit juices to change the taste of the protein drink.

7. Avoiding Poor Choices in the Kitchen

Good health is neither the denial of dieting nor the euphoria of eating.

The human canaries with battered bowel ecosystems do not tolerate sugars and starches well. Foods high in those substances feed the gut populations of "carb-loving" bacteria in their bowels and fan the fires of oxidative coagulopathy in their blood ecosystem and oxidative lymphopathy in their lymphatic ecosystem. Those changes markedly increase the detox burden in the liver ecosytem and lead to progressive oxidosis and dysoxygenosis. Thus, specific dietary measures taken to reverse various disease processes cannot be blindly recommended as optimal choices for healthful aging.

Good nutrition for healthful aging is common sense and the making of food choices that have stood the test of time. Modern science, in my view, helps us *understand* the mechanisms underlying the empirical observations of hundreds of generations that have gone before us. No studies conducted in mice or medical students for weeks or months must be allowed to negate the empirical experience of astute observers of the past centuries.

Martyrdom in the kitchen does not work. I cannot overstate the case for a sound philosophy of nutrition. Human canaries cannot eat well for a full life span except through a deep visceral-intuitive sense about how various foods affect their general level of energy and well-being. This cannot come from cortical obsessions about studying food charts and calorie tables. It requires a *learn-experiment-observe-learn* approach for adopting a *food philosophy.*

Specific plans for choices in the kitchen may be selected for addressing specific disorders, or even for different patterns of absence of health. For example, patients with damaged bowel ecology generally do better with food plans that comprise high-protein, high-fat (with emphasis on unoxidized fat) and low-carb food choices. Such plans prevent sugar roller coasters and insulin dysmetabolism. For those reasons, that diet plan is usually also effective for *short-term* programs for weight loss. I emphasize short-term here because, in my view, a high-fat, high-protein, no-starch diet probably carries more risk for more diseases than any other commonly used diet plan. Thus, from the standpoint of healthful aging, I do not recommend *long-term* use of high-fat, high-protein, no-carb diets.

Below, I provide a brief outline of essential nutritional issues for the September canaries.

1. Seek steady-state energy metabolism.
    - Avoid starving-gorging-starving cycles.
    - Avoid sugar-insulin-adrenaline roller coasters.
2. Maintain an optimal state of hydration.
    - Drink 50 to 70 ounces of high-compatibility fluids every day.
    - Drink fluids even when you are not thirsty.
3. Know your food reactivities.
    - Avoid foods that cause allergic reactions.
    - Avoid foods that deplete energy.
    - Avoid foods that cause abnormal bowel responses.
4. Focus on what you can eat.
    - De-focus foods that should be avoided.
    - Try new foods, observe their effects.
    - Think high-compatibility foods when food shopping.

5. Never miss breakfast.
    - Body tissues need to be energized in the morning.
    - Missing breakfast is fasting for 15 to 18 hours and sets us up for nutritional roller coasters.
    - Missing breakfast increases the need for undesirable stimulants such as coffee and tea.
6. Get the most out of vegetables.
    - Develop a taste for uncooked vegetables. (Taste is changeable.)
    - Develop a taste for steamed or stir-fried vegetables.
    - Reduce acidotic stress on metabolism. (Vegetables are alkaline-ash foods.)
7. Cut back on fruits.
    - Avoid allergenic fruits such as oranges.
    - Avoid very sweet fruits.
    - Avoid overripe fruits.
8. Increase proteins in food choices.
    - Proteins are time-release energy sources.
    - Proteins are building blocks for tissues and for energy and detoxification enzymes.
    - Minimize meat intake; increase lentils and beans.
9. Favor alkaline-ash foods.
    - Favor vegetables. (All biologic stressors increase acidotic stress. SAD [standard American diet] increases the body acid burden significantly.)
10. Minimize acid-ash foods.
    - Reduce intake of all meats.
    - Grains are, in general, acid-ash foods, but are needed to balance the alkalinity of vegetables and fruits.
11. Understand food cravings.
    - Food craving is the same thing as food addiction.

- Reduce salt intake.
- Reduce sugar intake.
- Eliminate or reduce intake of artificial sweeteners. (Salt, sugar and sweeteners increase sugar cravings.)

12. Have free access to healthful snacks.
    - The ideal snacks: uncooked or steamed vegetables.
    - Eat low-fructose fruits—those that are not very sweet.
    - Soynuts, pumpkin, sunflower and other seeds are also recommended.
    - Avoid walnuts and other tree nuts. (Tree nuts are among the most allergenic foods.)
13. Rotate foods.
    - High-compatibility foods may be eaten on three or less days a week.
    - Low-compatibility foods should not be eaten more often than once a week.
14. Ensure a healthy gut ecosystem.
    - Seed the bowel with healthful lactic acid-producing microbes.
    - Feed the lactic acid producers with nutrients such as pantothenic acid, vitamin B_{12}, fructose oligosaccharides and others.
    - Weed out the toxin-producing microbes such as yeasts, bacteria and parasites.
15. Eat limbically.
    - Follow visceral-intuitive impulses in making food choices. That, of course, is usually very difficult for those in the throes of sugar-insulin-adrenaline roller coasters. However, patience and persistence with these guidelines pays off.
    - Dieting plans are cortical traps.

    (Reading food labels becomes unnecessary after some time.)

16. Do not omit nutrient supplements.

- Take morning supplements with breakfast.
- Take evening supplements with dinner.
- Split daily supplements into three, four or more portions if problems of tolerance exist.
- Pollutants in the air can only be neutralized by nutrients.
- Contaminants in food can only be neutralized by nutrients.
- Toxins in water can only be neutralized by nutrients.

17. Don't be a skunk in someone's garden party by imposing your diet on others.

- It is not necessary.
- It is not desirable.
- Enzyme detoxification systems can cope with an occasional lapse—but only occasionally.

18. Bring some spiritual dimensions to your day.

- From extensive clinical work, I know that is the *single most* important matter in developing a long-term *livable* food philosophy. To reiterate what I wrote earlier, martyrdom doesn't work in nutrition. Good nutrition is neither the denial of dieting nor the euphoria of eating.

8. Relieving Constipation

I consider two to three effortless, odorless bowel movements every day an important criterion for health. Under physiological conditions, many changes occur throughout the gastrointestinal tract—including the mouth and the esophagus—that increase bowel motility and lead to evacuation. Thus, it is common for people in tribal cultures to have a bowel movement after almost every meal. Of course, there are no real lifestyle-related impediments to bowel evacuation in their lives. Many teachers consider that frequency of elimination simply impractical. Their teaching schedules make it difficult for them to respond immediately to their bowel signals with such frequency. I advise them to find two hours when they have free access to restrooms and overhydrate themselves in the beginning of that period.

Prolongation of the bowel transit time—with or without episodes of diarrhea—is very common in the human canaries. I try not to complete an office visit with any of them without ensuring that their bowel habit is regular and effective, or without taking some measures to achieve that. Of course, many of them report chronic constipation for years—some, in their words, all their lives. Years of neglect make the bowel very sluggish. Several of them were told, sometimes by their doctors, that it is normal for some people to have a bowel movement once every two or three days. Such statements amaze me. I wonder if engineers ever make similar statements about the exhaust systems of their machines.

The bowel is a dynamic, diverse, and delicate ecosystem. Dehydration and constipation are among two of the most important threats to the integrity of the bowel system. The bowel must not simply be seen as a dark, gurgling tube. It teems with life that can either preserve health or put it in jeopardy.

Most of the recommendations in the sections for optimal hydration and healthful choices in the kitchen restore bowel motility and prevent constipation. Uncooked vegetables are especially beneficial. Such measures are usually enough to relieve constipation and restore normal bowel motility in persons with occasional episodes of constipation. In general, certain vegetables—such as turnips, daikon, squashes, burdock, red radish, and green leafy vegetables—are very beneficial for preserving bowel health. Many people experience specific effects on the bowel transit time with specific uncooked vegetables and fruits. To learn about such food-bowel relationships, one needs to be aware of his bowel health and then observe. As I write this, I recall one patient who reported excellent bowel results with peaches and poor results, including staining of stools with blood, with mangoes.

What is food to one, is to others bitter poison.
Lucretius

The above primarily food-based approach may not be enough for persons with chronic and persistent constipation. Such individuals often have additional problems of adverse food reactions and unsuspected mold allergy that further diminish bowel motility. They require an integrated approach incorporating therapies including: (1) ample doses of magnesium, potassium, and taurine supplementation (doses used at the Institute are included later in the appendix); (2) natural substances, such as turkey rhubarb, triphala, cascara, and senna; (3) healthful microbes, such as *L. acidophilus* and *Bifidobacterium bifidus*; (4) judicious use of water, coffee, or sodium phosphate enemas; and (5) bowel detox protocols, such as colonic irrigations in selected cases. I make additional recommendations for restoring bowel ecology in the section dealing with that subject.

9. Avoiding Sugar-Insulin-Adrenaline Roller Coasters

Many people live lives in metabolic roller coasters without ever realizing the cause. Some live with sugar-insulin-adrenaline roller coasters, while others suffer adrenaline-cholinergic roller coasters. Many women live with PMS, wild mood swings and hot flushes caused by estrogen-progesterone-adrenaline roller coasters. Yet others are tormented by neurotransmitter roller coasters. In my clinical work, I consider elimination of such roller coasters as one of my primary goals.

Dysregulation of blood glucose level is a widespread problem in the United States. Below, I reproduce some text from *The Butterfly and Life Span Nutrition* to show how sugar roller coasters are produced.

> An eight-year-old child has a blood sugar level of 100 mg/dl (or 1,000 mg in one liter of blood). Since he has a total circulating blood volume of about 5 liters, the total quantity of glucose in his circulating blood is 5,000 mg or 5 grams. A teaspoonful of sugar holds 4 grams of sugar. Now this boy drinks a can of soda that contains 8 to 10 teaspoonfuls of sugar. This means that by drinking a can of soda, that child pours six to eight times as much sugar into his blood as exists at any time. Such a massive overload of sugar throws him into a sugar roller coaster, followed by an insulin roller coaster, which in turn triggers an adrenaline roller coaster. Similar molecular roller coasters are caused when he drinks a 12-ounce glass of commercial orange juice. How is the sugar molecular

> roller coaster initiated? With sugar overload. How is the sugar molecular roller coaster perpetuated? By withdrawal symptoms. "Highs" in the blood sugar levels are followed by the "lows" that create biologic demands for yet more sugar. Sugar craving is another name for sugar addiction. An American child at the turn of the century consumed between 5 and 10 pounds of sugar per year. His counterpart today ingests 150-175 pounds. How many thousands of molecular roller coasters does that come to? The numbers add up. This is the essence of the hypoglycemia problem. How does our sugar industry respond to all this? They keep physicians on their payroll to publish absurd studies showing that our children are not hurt by sugar. This is the simple truth behind the hypoglycemia controversy.

The best way to preserve the integrity of carbohydrate metabolism is to protect it from large and sudden sugar overloads. For this purpose, I strongly recommend breakfast comprised of suitable protein drinks containing eighty or higher percent calories in proteins and amino acids.

I protect the carbohydrate metabolism of my human canaries during afternoon and evening hours with prescriptions for supplemental cold-pressed essential oils to be taken cold. Specifically, I recommend that they take one to three tablespoons of one of the recommended oils an hour or so before dinner. The oil may be taken with steamed (and cooled) vegetables, salads, goat or sheep cheese, a small amount of grapefruit juice, or be simply taken as oil. My list of recommended oils includes extra virgin olive oil, flaxseed oil, sesame oil, avocado oil, grapeseed oil, pumpkin oil, safflower oil, almond oil and canola oil.

Ample but judicious prescriptions for vitamin and mineral supplements are needed for controlling metabolic roller coasters. I give my recommendations for this purpose later in the apendix.

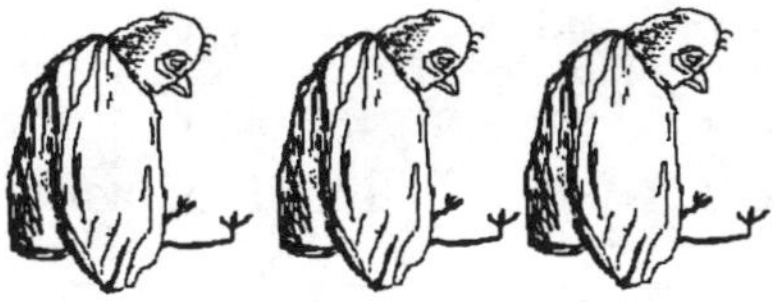

10. Managing Food Allergies and Incompatibilities

Food reactions are widely misunderstood. There are three important issues in understanding food allergy and sensitivity reactions: (1) allergy-causing genes; (2) frequency of consuming the food in question; and (3) the temperature of the *oxidative plate* of the body. In my clinical work, I find the last element to be most significant.

I introduced the concept of the oxidative plate in *The Canary and Chronic Fatigue* to emphasize the impact of the oxidative-dysoxygenative state in the body. I used the analogy of the hot plate in a popcorn machine. When the plate is cool, the corn put on it does not pop. When it is heated partially, some kernels will pop while others will not. When the plate is fully heated, nearly all kernels pop. I see the same phenomenon in my patients with fibromyalgia, chronic fatigue syndrome, and many chronic immune disorders. This phenomenon is sometimes called *spreading phenomenon.*

> In general, the sicker the person, the more frequent and troublesome the food reactions in food-sensitive individuals.

I see the reverse of that phenomenon when the general health of such patients improves with restorative oxygenative therapies. Their food reactions become fewer and less intense. When some of such patients relapse due to infections or chemical exposures, their food reactions become more frequent and intense. For advanced and professional readers, I have discussed this oxidative-dysoxygenative (OD) perspective of allergy elsewhere.

A source of confusion about food allergy and sensitivity reactions arises from failure to differentiate between *fixed* food allergy and *variable* food sensitivity reactions. The former is caused by a specific type of antibody called IgE antibodies and triggered by ingestion of a food against which such antibodies exist in the body. This type of reaction is fixed in the sense that every exposure to that food provokes a reaction. Such fixed food allergy can be reliably diagnosed by appropriate diagnostic skin test or micro-ELISA blood tests. The variable food reactions are more dependent on the state of the oxidative plate, i.e., the level of OD stress.

> The practical advice for the readers here is to learn to be *sensitive* to what is eaten and how that affects the state of their health. That may be possible by following the guidelines for eating and the tables giving lifespan and aging-oxidant food choices in the Appendix. For persons with chronic illnesses in which food reactions constitute significant clinical problems, it becomes necessary to work with a clinician experienced with food allergy and sensitivities.

11. Treating Mold (Yeast) Allergy

I think the "mold issue" is one of the most significant for the September canaries.

The mold issue—including the so-called yeast problem—has four faces: (1) IgE-mediated mold allergy; (2) overgrowth of PLFs in the bowel and blood; (3) mold toxins (mycotoxins); and (4) mold (yeast) infections.

Mold allergy and toxicity are among the most important causes of chronic illness. It is noteworthy that in true desert communities, serious chronic immune disorders such as multiple sclerosis, rheumatoid arthritis, lupus, scleroderma and vasculitis are virtually unknown. In my view, this is largely due to the fact that molds require closed, humid and dark places to flourish and such places are rare in deserts. Reduction of exposure to molds—also called yeasts—is of central importance in successful management of inhalant allergy. Pollens are in the air for limited periods of time; mold spores are in the air throughout the year in most instances. It is not possible to eliminate mold exposure altogether. I reproduce here some text from my monograph, *Allergy: Diagnosis and Management*, to provide some guidelines for reducing exposure to mold:

1. Humidity levels at home should be kept low—in summer below 35% if possible with the air conditioner or dehumidifier. Minimize the use of humidifiers in the winter.
2. Exhaust fans should be used in the bathroom and above the stove when cooking.
3. Visible mildew and other molds in the home should be removed with nontoxic solutions. A solution of two tablespoons of baking soda in one cup of vinegar and one pint

of water may be used to remove visible deposits of mold. An alternative cleansing solution is to use equal parts of household bleach and water for this purpose.

4. Heavy leather items should not be kept in the bedroom.
5. The number of mold-breeding indoor plants should be kept low. Molds grow well in indoor planters.
6. Some long-term measures include substituting paints for wallpaper. Heavy drapes should be avoided, and heavy garments and sleeping bags should not be piled on the floor of closets.
7. Prolonged periods of time in dark and humid (moldy) areas should be avoided, such as basements, attics, barns, and areas with decomposing grass and compost.
8. Discretion should be used during extended hiking in woods or working on lawns in the height of pollen season if you suffer from pollen allergy. (Pollen exposure will increase mold sensitivity in this setting.)
9. Discretion should be exercised in visiting antique shops, old book shops and other such areas where molds flourish.

Foods that may trigger allergic reactions in mold-sensitive canaries are: fermented foods (especially beer and wine), vinegar and salad dressings, aged cheeses, malt and foods containing malt, dried fruits, mushrooms, peanuts and peanut butter, and pickles and pickled foods. Another issue is that of toxins produced by molds. In general, the longer the time yeasts have to grow in foods, the greater the risk of toxicity with mold toxins. Thus yeast in baked bread does not have the same risk as yeast in fermented foods.

The practical advice for the readers here is to learn to be *aware* of relevant mold exposures and how such exposures affect their state of health. For persons with chronic illnesses in which mold allergy reactions constitute significant clinical problems, it becomes necessary to work with a clinician experienced with mold allergy and sensitivities.

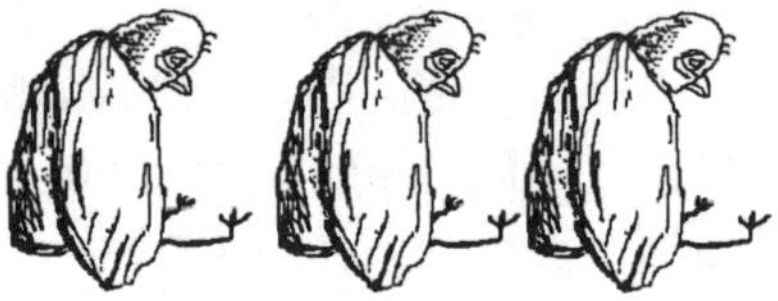

The human immune system is rooted in the soil of the bowel.

12. Reducing Environmental (Chemical) Sensitivities

Chemical sensitivity is dose independent, while chemical toxicity is dose related. I made that critical distinction earlier. The failure to appreciate this critical difference by doctors led to mistreatment of many September canaries.

During the last twenty-five years, there have been great advances in understanding allergic reactions. And yet, *certain basic questions about such reactions remain unanswered.* For example, skin allergy conditions, such as eczema lesions, flare more in some weeks than in others in the same person. Lifestyle stressors cause more wheezing on some days than on others in the same asthma sufferer. Abdominal cramps, bloating, and diarrhea in Crohn's colitis and ulcerative colitis ease off or intensify for no apparent reason in most persons with those conditions. Food sensitivity reactions vary over a broad range in the same individual. Nasal and sinus congestion become more intense on some days when pollen count is low and abate on days when pollen counts are high. This spreading phenomenon is increasingly recognized in chronic fatigue syndrome, fibromyalgia, and multiple chemical sensitivity syndrome. The molecular cause of none of the above can be understood on the basis of the classical knowledge of allergy. Those considerations led me to look beyond the matter of allergy caused by IgE antibodies and put forth an oxidative-dysoxygenative disorder as the molecular model for human canaries. All mediator responses of allergy are greatly amplified by oxidative coagulopathy and its cellular consequences. The clinical symptoms of allergy in the September canaries had to be seen as the visible tip of a much larger iceberg of foundational changes in the trio of the bowel, blood, and liver ecosystems.

During the past few decades, a wide gulf developed between the views of university-based allergy researchers and clinical ecologists (physicians who focused on *clinically verifiable* patterns of hypersensitivity reactions that can be explained neither on the basis of IgE antibodies nor with any of the other recognized immunologic sensitivity mechanisms). The core concepts of clinical ecology included the following: (1) total load; (2) sensitization; (3) maladaptation; and (4) deadaptation. In the author's own opinion, the classical view of atopy simply could not explain a broad spectrum of clinical manifestations of hypersensitivity responses. The academicians continued to focus on effects of injection therapy with single allergens, such as cat dander or ragweed. The ecologists, while recognizing the theoretical value of such work, found such observations of very limited value to the care of the ill, who invariably suffered multiple sensitivities. After decades of doubt and denial, the existence of multiple chemical sensitivity syndrome was finally acknowledged and its relevance to the management of classical allergy understood.

13. Correcting Functional Nutritional Deficiencies.

Nutritional status is impoverished in many Americans. My colleagues and I perform laboratory assessments of the body reserves of essential vitamins, minerals, and other natural redox-active nutrients in all patients with chronic disorders. It is uncommon for us to find persons who show levels of such nutrients within a healthy range. For example, a 24-hour urine mineral analysis which we conduct routinely on all patients nearly always reveals deficiencies of essential minerals as well as excesses of toxic metals. This is also true in most patients who consult us for disorders that are commonly *not* considered to be associated with nutrient deficiencies, including coronary artery disease, stroke, Alzheimer's disease, arthritis, vasculitis, and others.

A Single Robber Goes Down With Six Cops

Our nutrition is in jeopardy for many reasons. The prevalent use of highly processed foods, sugar overload, and regular exposure to preservatives and pesticide residues in food items creates many *functional* nutritional deficiencies. I often use the following analogy to explain why functional nutritional deficiencies are so common today. Suppose the people in a town are deeply troubled by a high rate of robberies in their houses and the frequent escape of robbers from the town prison. In their frustration, they establish a strict rule that whenever a cop catches a robber, the cop will also stay in the prison cell handcuffed to the robber. That may seem irrational, but that is exactly how the cops-and-robbers game is played in the human body. Robbers are the synthetic chemical poisons and toxic metabolic waste substances. Cops are the nutrients. The toxic molecules (robbers) are literally trapped by the nutrient molecules (cops) and both stay bound to each other.

Then I extend the analogy. The town people learn of a big tragedy. They are shocked to find out that the robbers again escaped the prison, but took along the cops handcuffed to them. A fight broke out among the cops and robbers and they shot and killed each other. Something very close to that happens in human detox pathways. Sometimes as many as six molecules of glutathione (an especially good detox cop) are bound to some pesticide (a particularly nasty robber) and are wasted by the kidney. *Six cops wasted for every robber gotten rid of!*

This nutrient-toxin relationship is not fully appreciated by many doctors who question the value of nutrient supplementation in integrative medicine. Such doctors often ask for proof that functional nutritional deficiencies indeed do exist. My colleagues and I see the proof of that every working day when patients report recovery from fibromyalgia and disabling fatigue after such therapies. Furthermore, on many occasions when our patients discontinue their nutrient supplementation, their symptoms recur. We also document the biochemical evidence of their value by appropriate laboratory tests.

In the table below, I furnish some general information about vitamins, minerals, and other redox-restorative substances which my colleagues and I prescribe for our patients.

Table 3. General Guidelines for Nutrient Supplementation for the September Canaries

	Early Cases of the September Eleven Syndrome	Advanced Cases of the September Eleven Syndrome
Vitamins	Vitamins: C, 1,000 to 2,000 mg; E, 200 to 400 IU; A, 5,000 to 7,500 IU; D, 100 to 250 IU; B-complex, 25-50 mg; B12, 1,000 mcg weekly for four weeks.	Vitamins: C, 3,000 to 5,000 mg; E, 400 to 800 IU; A, 10,000 to 15,000 IU; D, 100 to 250 IU; B-complex, 30-50 mg; B12, 1,000 to 5,000 mcg weekly for four to six weeks.
Minerals	Magnesium, 1,000 to 1,500 mg; Calcium, 1,000 to 1,500 mg; Potassium, 200 to 400 mg; Chromium, 50-100 mcg; Selenium, 50-100 mcg; Molybdenum, 50-100 mcg.	Magnesium, 1,500 to 2,500 mg; Calcium, 1,000 to 1,500 mg; Potassium, 400 to 600 mg; Chromium, 200-400 mcg; Selenium, 200-400 mcg; Molybdenum, 200-400 mcg.
Redox-Restorative Substances	Glutathione, 200-300 mg; N-acetylcysteine, 200-300 mg; MSM (Methylsulfonylmethane) 200-500 mg; Lipoic acid, 100 to 200 mg; Taurine, 500 to 1,000 mg; Coenzyme Q10, 30 to 50 mg; Pycnogenol, 50 to 100 mg.	Glutathione, 600-800 mg; N-acetylcysteine, 600-800 mg; MSM, 500 to 1,500 mg; Lipoic acid, 100 to 500 mg; Taurine, 500 to 1,500 mg; Coenzyme Q10, 100-150 mg; Pycnogenol, 100 to 150 mg.

14. Balancing Hormones

From the standpoint of hormonal imbalance in the September canaries, the following are the important issues:

1. Hormones are molecular messengers.
2. Hormones play many and *varying* roles in the web of life.
3. When one hormone system is changed in one way, something is changed in every other hormone system. Hormones turn into each other according to the prevailing cellular ecologic conditions.
4. Hormones are essential to *every* cellular function, and not just the limited roles that are assigned to them in medical texts.
5. Disruptions of the base trio of the bowel, blood, and liver ecosystems are at the root of problems such as premenstrual syndrome (PMS), endometriosis, and menstrual irregularities (including loss of menstruation in young women with fibromyalgia, chronic fatigue syndrome, and chemical sensitivity syndrome).
6. The epidemic of breast cancer, in my view, is directly linked to the avalanche of synthetic hormones that children and adults are exposed to in their daily lives.
7. *All* hormone systems are essential for healthful aging; however, no single hormone or prehormone can be used for extending the lifespan.

Some readers are likely to raise their eyebrows on my assertion that menstrual disorders are related to battered bowel, blood, and liver ecosystems. My colleagues at the Institute and I published the evidence for that view in a clinical outcome study of young women with fibromyalgia and CFS who also reported oligomenorrhea (fewer or scanty periods) and amenorrhea (complete loss of menstruation). Their menstrual functions were completely or nearly completely restored by our integrative plans with focus on restorative and oxygenative therapies that *primarily* addressed issues of those ecosystems.

Others might be surprised by my statement that epidemics of breast and prostate cancers are due to exposure to synthetic hormones. I state my case simply. Consider the incidence of those two cancers in different regions of the globe during the last century. You will note that widespread use of synthetic hormones and xenoestrogens (pesticides and related chemicals with estrogen-like effects) in all countries was followed by rising incidences of those two cancers. Both cancers were distinctly uncommon among the Japanese prior to World War II, and became increasingly common during the post-war decades as the population was increasingly exposed to synthetic hormones and pesticides. China today makes for an illuminating study of that phenomenon. In the wealthy big cities of eastern China (Beijing, Shanghai, Nanjing, and others), the incidence of both cancers is rising. In the rural and poor populations of western China, those cancers are still uncommon.

For restoring hormonal equilibrium in the September canaries, I focus heavily on all relevant issues of the bowel, blood, and liver ecosystems. Next, based on appropriate laboratory test results, I offer an integrated program employing natural substances that support hormone ecosystems, such as licorice, wild yam, dong quai, black and blue cohosh, false unicorn root, fennel and sarsaparilla. Sometimes I use a "layered" approach that includes such substances as DHEA, pregnenolone, androstenedione, and others. Most September canaries show abnormalities in their blood and urine tests and it becomes necessary to prescribe hormones derived from soybean and other natural sources.

The practical advice for the reader here is to learn the importance of *all* hormone systems for healthful aging of *all* cellular and tissue-organ ecosystems of the body, and not merely for improving sexual function or controlling menopausal symptoms. I strongly recommend that readers resist the temptation of taking any hormone or prehormone for preserving health without the direct and *ongoing supervision* of an experienced clinician.

15. Reducing Toxic Metal Overload

A California dentist consulted me for severe rheumatoid arthritis and debilitating fatigue, which forced her to stop work several months before I saw her. She had been a vigorous person who worked 50 to 60 hours a week and then had energy to live an active social life. She had no prior symptoms of joint or muscle pain. A doctor had performed a urine mercury test following a test dose of DMPS (a potent mercury chelator). The next day she did not feel well. Within a few days, she developed progressive generalized joint stiffness and pain and increasing fatigue. Within weeks she was totally disabled. Since that case, I have seen other similar examples of serious illness caused by acute mercury toxicity resulting from rapid mercury chelation with DMPS.

A young woman with multiple sclerosis suffered from progressive muscle stiffness and pain, numbness in limbs, urinary difficulties, and increasing fatigue. She responded well to our integrative program and within several months was completely symptom free. A urine mineral profile performed after an intravenous dose of 1.5 grams of EDTA (a very weak mercury chelator) revealed raised levels of mercury and some other toxic metals. She wanted to have mercury fillings in her teeth replaced with composite ones. I agreed with her, since she had been stable and free of any signs of the disease for several months. With additional nutrient support, we cautiously began the process and scheduled one removal session every two months. *After each such session she missed her next menstrual cycle.* Several months following the last session, at the age of 29, she conceived her first child.

Heavy metal overload and toxicity are widely misunderstood areas. Except for integrative physicians and clinical ecologists, doctors rarely, if ever, order tests for 24-hour urine or blood levels of toxic metals, such as mercury, lead, aluminum, cadmium, and arsenic. Hence, the problem, when it exists, remains undiagnosed and ignored. Pediatricians who diligently look for lead overload in children often find clear evidence for that. Integrative physicians who routinely order mineral analysis for their patients fully recognize how widespread heavy metal toxicity is in Americans.

The clinical pictures of acute heavy metal toxicities are well characterized and generally described at length in medical textbooks. What is rarely, if ever, addressed in those texts is the critical issue of *cumulative* toxic metal burden in persons compromised with chronic nutritional, immune and ecologic disorders. Of course, that further feeds the fires of dissent in this important area.

In the context of oxygen and aging, it is noteworthy that many toxic metals inflict heavy damage on antioxidant enzyme systems of the body. For example, mercury rips apart the sulfhydryl bonds in such redox-essential substances as glutathione.

16. Diminishing Synthetic Chemical Overload

Three things come to my mind as I begin this section. First, during summer months, we occasionally lost air conditioning in our hospital laboratory for several hours. At such times, the test results obtained with some equipment showed mild elevations in the enzyme activities in the blood samples of some patients. In the chemistry section, some staff members also experienced irritability, headaches, and related problems.

Second, one of my associate pathologists examined biopsies and surgical specimens sent to the laboratory in formalin (formaldehyde) on Tuesdays and Fridays. Sometimes emergencies and conference and vacation schedules forced her to do such work on two consecutive days. She often developed a headache on the evening of the second day.

Third, formaldehyde is a very strong irritant, a common cause of chemical sensitivity, and a carcinogen in animals. The law required that we monitor exposure of our staff in the histology section (where they worked with formaldehyde all the time). So they carried formaldehyde sensors during work hours. We were all very sensitive to the issue and used multiple specially exhausted air filter systems there. While establishing the monitoring mechanism, on an impulse I asked the laboratory manager to get one control person in our personnel department to also wear the formaldehyde monitor for a comparative study of exposures. He smiled and accepted my challenge, humoring my eccentricity, I'm sure. He came to my office some weeks later, laughing and holding the survey reports. The results showed that the person in the personnel department had a greater exposure to formaldehyde than *any* of the laboratory staff! We realized that the air in the personnel department without special air filters actually contained more fomaldehyde than in the laboratory.

Three Issues of Chemical Overload

There are three core issues in the matter of synthetic chemicals and healthful aging: (1) *cumulative* body burden of synthetic chemicals; (2) *cumulative* toxicity of chemicals; and (3) *cumulative* cellular functional and structural damage caused by chemicals.

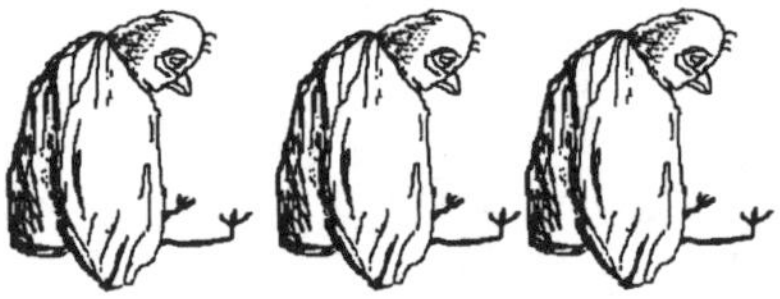

Cumulative Burden of Synthetic Chemicals

As for cumulative chemical burden, it is estimated that Americans are exposed to nearly 65,000 synthetic chemicals in their daily lives. The liver, as indicated previously, is the first-line-of-defense organ for most such chemicals. Even though the liver has

Cumulative Burden of Synthetic Chemicals

As for cumulative chemical burden, it is estimated that Americans are exposed to nearly 65,000 synthetic chemicals in their daily lives. The liver, as indicated previously, is the first-line-of-defense organ for most such chemicals. Even though the liver has enormous functional reserves, it cannot eliminate or detoxify *all* such substances, so their accumulation begins. Many synthetic chemicals are fat soluble and have a greater affinity for brain tissue than many other tissues. Having gained entry into the brain, such chemicals are not in any hurry to leave. Indeed, they *accumulate* there for years. Those facts explain why chemical detox plans give delayed results.

Cumulative Toxicity of Synthetic Chemicals

My father, a judge, used to say that one and one in a court of law do not make two. Sometimes we get 11. That, it seems to me, happens more often to synthetic chemicals in the body than in the courts of law. Many chemicals not only add to the toxicity of other chemicals, they also *amplify* each other's toxic effects. Of special relevance to the present discussion are the oxidative-dysoxygenative *chain* reactions that are triggered by synthetic chemicals and involve fats, proteins, sugars, enzymes, cell receptors, and DNA in the body. Again, I emphasize the *cumulative* aspect of the above processes.

Cumulative Cellular Damage Caused by Chemicals

There is a wide gulf on this subject among academics and clinical ecologists. The academics rarely, if ever, assess the *functional* consequences of chemicals on the human body. Their studies are largely limited to effects of exposures of small animals to large doses of chemicals—they use terms like minimum lethal dose to characterize the toxicity of the chemical. Such an approach is *fundamentally* irrelevant to the subject of functional and structural cellular changes caused by chemicals.

Blood and urine tests for measuring chemical overload are routinely performed by many clinical ecologists. However, the state of the art seriously limits their efforts. Evidence for such toxicity is amply clear to clinicians who undertake slow and steady detox programs for their patients with ecologic and immune disorders.

I believe the *cumulative* threat posed by chemicals to human health is a very serious issue which is rarely, if ever, addressed by the main physician body in the United States.

17. Cleansing the Bowel

The bowel ecosystem *is* the foundation of the pyramid of human ecosystems. Readers by now should be familiar with the experimental and clinical evidence I present in this book to support that view. It should not come as a surprise that I consider measures taken to preserve the integrity of the bowel ecosystem in health and its restoration in disease as *fundamental* to the goal of aging healthfully. Below, I adapt some text from my monograph, *Altered States of Bowel Ecology,* first published in 1987.

The Seed, Feed, and Occasionally Weed Approach

An integrated *seed, feed, and occasionally weed* approach is the centerpiece of *all* my attempts for preserving the bowel ecology for healthful aging, as well as for restoring bowel ecosystems battered by antibiotic abuse and sugar overload.

Seeding is the repopulation of the bowel ecosystem with microbes that normally preserve it. I call such microbes guardian angels of human health. It is necessary because our bowel ecology is under unrelenting assault by antibiotics fed to our poultry and cattle, as well as those prescribed by doctors. Another important factor is sugar overload. Both factors lead to overgrowth of oxygen-hating, acid-loving primordial life forms (PLFs) in the bowel that literally crowd out the healthful microbes.

Feeding is the use of growth factors required by the healthful bowel microbes, such as *Bifidobacterium bifida* and *Lactobacillus acidophilus*. Those growth factors include vitamin B_{12}, pantothenic acid, biotin, and others. I do not think it is coincidental that both vitamin B_{12} and pantothenic acid are essential for the health of humans as well as their guardian-angel microbes.

Occasional weeding is accomplished by the use of several natural substances that suppress the overgrowth of PLFs, as well as viruses and disease-causing bacteria. The best known—and the most widely used worldwide—is plain yogurt. However, that may not be enough to prevent damage to the bowel ecology caused by antibiotics.

Table 4. Therapies for Restoring the Battered Bowel Ecosystem

For healthy persons:
Water therapies
Organic vegetable juices
Bowel-friendly vegetables
Optimal choices in the kitchen
Freshly fileted aloe
Ginger/garlic
Magnesium, potassium, and taurine
Psyllium husk and apple pectin

For persons with history of bowel disorders:
Vitamin B_{12}
Pantothenic acid and pantetheine
Fennel seeds, fenugreek, licorice, and pau d' Arco
Echinacea, astragalus, goldenseal, and burdock root
Grape seed extract
Oral hydrogen peroxide
Coffee, water, and probiotic enemas
Hydrogen peroxide baths
Colon hydrotherapy
Diagnosis and management of food sensitivities and mold allergy

The exact formulations for 14 bowel protocols are given in the Appendix.

18. Cleansing the Blood

I consider the bloodstream as an ecosystem sandwiched between the other two great ecosystems of the body: the bowel and liver ecosystems. Next to the bowel, oxygenative therapies that address *all* issues of the blood ecology are the most effective treatments for acute and subacute disorders. Such therapies also rank high among my priorities for healthful aging. Furthermore, it will be obvious to the reader by now that, in my view, a drop of blood smeared on a slide provides us the *best window to the world of human biology*, including the matters of healthful aging and disease.

Table 5. Therapies for Restoring the Polluted Blood Ecosystem
Nasal oxygen
Oral hydrogen peroxide
Hydrogen peroxide bath
Intravenous hydrogen peroxide infusion
Intravenous ozone infusion
Intravenous EDTA infusion
Intravenous nutrient infusions
Intramuscular infusion
Mercury and other toxic metal chelation

As is the case with nutrient therapies, doctors unfamiliar with the therapies listed in the above table frequently make derisive comments about treatment methods. For those who wish to directly assess the efficacy of such therapies, I suggest simple examination of blood smears of the patient before and after such therapies are administered. They will quickly recognize what my colleagues and I see every working day.

> A drop of blood smeared on a slide and seen with a high-resolution microscope provides the *best window* to the state of oxidation and oxygenation of the person.

The blood smears of the September canaries become much *cleaner* after effective detox, antioxidant, and oxygenative therapies.

19. Detoxifying the Liver

Next to the bowel, the liver is the most important guardian angel of oxygen metabolism. I support that view with several lines of evidence and my personal observations in my book, *Oxygen and Aging*. Thus, I believe the liver, next to the bowel, must be the focus for all oxygenative and antioxidant therapies for reversing dysoxygenosis and preserving health. For emphasis, I again point out that all therapies that primarily address issues of the bowel and blood ecosystems also restore the liver ecosystem and health.

In Table 6, I list therapies that my colleagues and I prescribe for restoring the damaged liver ecosystem.

Table 6. Liver Detox Therapies

Therapies that normalize cellular oxygen metabolism by focusing on restoration of the bowel, blood, and liver ecosystems include the following:

1. Liver-protective foods, such as ginger, garlic, onions, black radish, turmeric, beets, turnips, burdock, dandelion, and others;
2. Liver-friendly nutrients, such as inositol, choline, lecithin, methionine, glutathione, N-acetylcysteine, MSM, lipoic acid, and others;
3. Liver-friendly herbs, such as aloe, milk thistle, catnip, goldenseal, red clover, fennel seeds, Jerusalem artichoke, and others;
4. Liver and gall bladder flush;
5. Liver castor oil packs;
6. Kidney flush;
7. All measures taken to prevent chemical overload on the liver as well as all therapies designed to reduce total chemical overload.

I refer the advanced and professional readers to *Integrative Medicine: The Principles and Practice* for detailed descriptions and discussion of the above therapies and procedures.

The exact formulations for two liver protocols are given in the Appendix. These protocols include liver-friendly nutrients and herbs that my colleagues and I prescribe for our patients with chronic disorders characterized by liver congestion and enlargement with or without elevated blood activities of enzymes (which indicate the presence of liver injury). We also employ those protocols for all patients with various types of viral hepatitis.

Liver Castor Oil Pack and Liver Flush Protocol

Two natural therapies that have stood the test of time for liver detoxification are liver castor oil pack and liver flush protocols. As for other specific therapies I include in this book, I recommend that both liver pack and flush should be undertaken under professional supervision first. I myself prescribe castor oil liver packs to facilitate liver detox and reduce liver congestion as a part of our basic bowel-blood-liver detox program in most patients with chronic ailments. Both protocols are included in the Appendix of this book.

The practical advice here is to undertake liver detoxification under the supervision of a clinician experienced in this area.

20. Intramuscular and Intravenous Nutrient and Oxygenative Therapies

In preparing my guidelines for the prevention and reversal of the September Eleven syndrome, I have been mindful both of the wisdom of the ancients and modern science. It is amazing how closely the latter has validated the former. Indeed, in many ways, my work may be seen as an effort to develop as well as marshal experimental and modern clinical evidence to support the ancient healing philosophies. *Moderation, the ancients counseled, was the best strategy in eating*. That, in essence, is one of the messages of this chapter. *Know thyself*, they also advised. That is another important message. To me, *knowing oneself* means how one can move towards *one's own* spiritual surrender, *one's own* freedom from confused demands of love and anger, *one's own sense* of sanctity of his environment, and *one's own sense* of right food choices. The ancients understood—intuitively, it seems to me—that diseases of the body are rooted in the bowel. I came to the same conclusion after the study of over 14,000 bowel and 5,000 stomach biopsies, and after caring for over 5,000 patients with nutritional, ecologic, immunologic, and degenerative disorders.

Earlier I expressed my disillusionment with the gurus of the weight-loss industry. The issue is not whether some of those diets can help some people lose weight some of the time—or that weight loss is not desirable for many Americans. The real issue in the context of healthful aging is this: Weight loss that ruins metabolism cannot promote healthful aging.

Two lead articles in a recent issue of *The New England Journal of Medicine* told us that fiber and low-fat diets (factors that promote health) do not reduce the incidence of colon polyps. *That is bad science* because it only indicates *bad study design* that fails to take into account the diversity, dynamics, and delicacy of the bowel ecosystem. There is no substitute for learning, trying, observing, and knowing.

My colleagues and I prescribe intramuscular and intravenous nutrient protocols primarily for two objectives:

1. To overcome the problem of poor intestinal absorption commonly seen in the September Eleven syndrome; and
2. To create a large gradient for nutrients across the cell membranes in order to facilitate their entry into cells.

We employ intravenous oxygen therapies, such as hydrogen peroxide infusions and ozone, to normalize oxygen metabolism because at this time there are no effective oral programs for that.

In general, most patients require four to eight intravenous treatments or ten to 16 intramuscular injections to reach a stage in which oral nutrient protocols begin to provide the desired support. In the tables given below, I furnish compositions of some of the intramuscular and intravenous protocols which my colleagues and I commonly prescribe for human canaries. We established the long-term safety of those protocols with extensive clinical outcome studies.

Professional and advanced readers can obtain detailed information about those protocols from www.aginghealthfully.com.

INTRAMUSCULAR 1 PROTOCOL		
Nutrient	Concentration	Volume
Magnesium sulfate	500 mg/ml	1.5 ml
Calcium gly/lac	10 mg/ml	1.5 ml
Vitamin B_{12}	1,000 mcg/ml	1 ml
Vit. B complex	*	1 ml
Pantothenic acid	250 mg/ml	0.5 ml
Pyridoxin	100 mg/ml	0.5 ml
Zinc	5 mg/ml	0.6 ml
Molybdenum	25 mcg/ml	0.5 ml
Selenium	40 mcg/ml	0.4 ml
Multivitamins	**	0.5 ml

* Vitamin B complex includes the following per ml: thiamine, 100 m; riboflavin, 2 mg; niacinamide, 100 mg; dexpanthenol, 2 mg; pyridoxine, 2 mg.
**Multivitamin solution contains: Vit. A, 10,000 IU; Vit. D, 1,000 IU; thiamin HCI, 50 mg; riboflavin, 10 mg; pyridoxine HCI, 15 mg; niacinamide, 100 mg; dexpanthenol, 25 mg; Vit. E 5 IU.

INTRAMUSCULAR 2 PROTOCOL		
Nutrient	Concentration	Volume
Magnesium sulfate	500 mg/ml	3 ml
Calcium gly/lac	10 mg/ml	3.5 ml
Vitamin B_{12}	1,000 mcg/ml	1.5 ml

INTRAMUSCULAR 5 PROTOCOL		
Nutrient	Concentration	Volume
Magnesium sulfate	500 mg/ml	1.5 ml
Calcium gly/lac	10 mg/ml	1.5 ml
Vitamin B_{12}	10,000 mcg/ml	1 ml
Vit B. complex	*	0.5 ml
Pantothenic acid	250 mg/ml	0.5 ml
Pyridoxine	100 mg/ml	0.5 ml
Zinc	5 mg/ml	0.6 ml
Molybdenum	25 mcg/ml	0.5 ml
Selenium	40 mcg/ml	0.4 ml
Multivitamins	**	0.5 ml

INTRAMUSCULAR 6 PROTOCOL		
Nutrient	Concentration	Volume
Magnesium sulfate	500 mg/ml	3 ml
Calcium gly/lac	10 mg/ml	4 ml
Vitamin B_{12}	10,000 mcg/ml	0.5 ml

* Vitamin B complex includes the following per ml: thiamine, 100 m; riboflavin, 2 mg; niacinamide, 100 mg; dexpanthenol, 2 mg; pyridoxine, 2 mg.
**Multivitamin solution contains: Vit. A, 10,000 IU; Vit. D, 1,000 IU; thiamin HCI, 50 mg; riboflavin, 10 mg; pyridoxine HCI, 15 mg; niacinamide, 100 mg; dexpanthenol, 25 mg; Vit. E 5 IU.

INTRAVENOUS OXIDATIVE STRESS PROTOCOL	
Vitamin C	20 gm
Vitamin A	6,600 IU
Vitamin D	400 IU
Vitamin E	20 IU
Biotin	120 mcg
Folic acid	800 mcg
Niacinamide	80 mg
Riboflavin	7.2 mg
Thiamine	6 mg
Pantothenic acid	530 mg
Pyridoxine	108 mg
Cyanocobalamine*	2,500 mcg
Taurine	50 mg
Calcium gluconate	125 mg
Copper sulfate	3.2 mg
Chromium	32 mcg
Magnesium sulfate	2,000 mg
Manganese	0.8 mg
Molybdenum	100 mcg
Zinc sulfate	24 mg
Selenium	200 mcg
Taurine	50 mg

*Cyanocobalamine is given as an IM injection (1ml)

Administration Time
2-1/2 to 3 hours

INTRAVENOUS CHELATION PROTOCOL (EDTA DOSE 1.5 GM)	
EDTA (disodium)	1.5 gm
Vitamin C	5 gm
Magnesium sulfate	2,000 mg
Pantothenic Acid	500 mg
Pyridoxine	200 mg
Cyanocobalamine	1,500 mcg
Vitamin A	3,300 IU
Vitamin D	200 IU
Vitamin E	10 IU
Biotin	60 mcg
Folic acid	400 mcg
Niacinamide	40 mg
Riboflavin	3.6 mg
Thiamine	3 mg
Pyridoxine	4 mg
Pantothenic acid	15 mg
Sodium bicarbonate	1.25 mEq
Procaine 2%	30 mg
Heparin (5,000 units/cc)	2,000 U

Solution

Ringer's lactate, 250 ml

Administration Time

1-1/2 to 2 hours

Preparation

As for Chelation I Protocol except for the EDTA dose of

EDTA, disodium salt	7 ml
Magnesium sulfate	4 ml
Pyridoxine	2 ml
Pantothenic acid	2 ml
Vitamin C	10 ml
Multi-vitamin	10 ml
Heparin (5,000U/ml)	0.4 ml
Procaine 2%	1.5 ml
Sodium bicarbonate	2.5 ml

Other

Vitamin B_{12} (1,000 mcg) is given separately with an IM injection at the end of each chelation.

Solution

Ringer's lactate, 150 ml

Administration Time

2 hours

INTRAVENOUS HYDROGEN PEROXIDE PROTOCOL
(to be administered in two parts)

H_2O_2 PART A		
Nutrient	Concentration=Volume	Amount
Hydrogen peroxide	3.75%	0.35 ml
Sodium bicarbonate	0.5 mEq/ml=1.25 mEq	2.5 ml
Normal saline		150 ml
NUTRIENTS PART B		
Magnesium sulfate	500 mg/ml = 1.5 ml	750 mg
Zinc	5 mg/ml =2 ml	12 mg
Calcium gly/lac	10 mg/ml =7.5 ml	75 mg
Pantothenic acid	250 mg/ml =1.5 ml	375 mg
Pyridoxine	100 mg/ml =1 ml	100 mg
Vitamin C	500 mg/ml =1 ml	0.5 gm
Vitamin B complex	See table 4	1 ml
Molybdenum	25 mcg/ml = 5 ml	125 mcg
Taurine	50 mg/ml = 2 ml	100 mg
Glutathione	60 mg/ml = 2 ml	120 mg
Vitamin B12	1000 mcg = 1 ml	1000 mcg
Sodium bicarbonate	2.5 m Eq/5 ml=1.5 ml	------
Lidocaine	20 mg/ml = 1.5 ml	30 mg
0.9% normal saline		100 ml

Health depends on whether or not the body's self-cleansing mechanisms can cope with the *total* body burden of metabolic and environmental toxins that lead to oxidosis, acidosis, and dysoxygenosis.

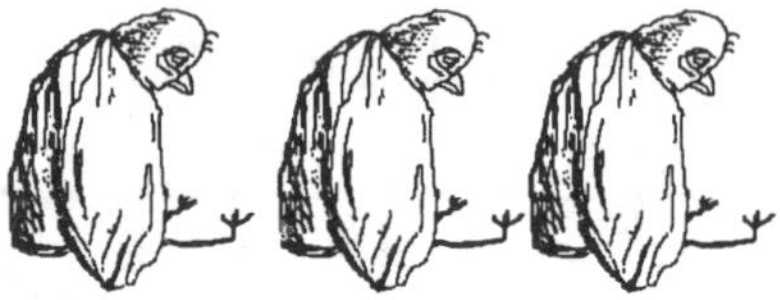

In closing, prevention and treatment of the September Eleven syndrome requires a holistic and integrative philosophy. The problem of oxygen dysfunction in this syndrome is global. And so must be the treatment philosophy.

The victim of the syndrome and his physician both need a gardener's sense of nurturing—of seeding, feeding, watering, and occasionally weeding the ecosystems of the body. The blocker drugs —beta blockers, channel blockers, enzyme inhibitors, suppressor of mediators of healing, drugs that inactivate various cellular pumps—are often necessary for temporary control of symptoms. But, there must be no illusions about drugs being the *real* treatment. There are no drugs that normalize a dysfunctional oxygen metabolism.

Appendix

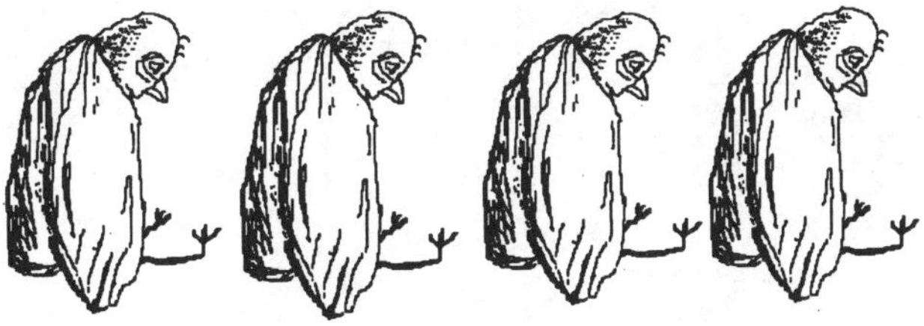

AGING HEALTHFULLY FOOD CHOICES

BEVERAGES	PROTEINS	FATS
1st Choice	1st Choice	1st Choice
Carbon-filtered water Fresh vegetable juice Ginger water Banch tea Grain coffee Herbal teas Spring water Deep well water	Protein Peptide powders Hunted fish Lentils Beans Duck Quail Wild game Goat Sheep Lamb Guinea hen Muscovy duck Whole grains Spirolina Plankton	Olive oil Ghee Butter Sesame oil Flaxseed oil
2nd Choice	2nd Choice	2nd Choice
Bottled spring water Bottled deep well water Mineral water Fruit teas Grapefruit juice Apple juice Soy milk, diluted Rice milk, diluted Sheep's milk Goat's milk Buffalo's milk Green teas	Chicken Turkey Shellfish Cornish hen Egg	Safflower oil Sunflower oil Soybean oil Avocado oil Canola oil
3rd Choice	3rd Choice	3rd Choice
Skim milk, cow Low-fat cow's milk Light diet sodas Grape juice Cranberry juice Orange juice Coconut juice Nut milks, diluted Salted vegetable juice	Beef Veal Pork Cultured fish	Corn oil Cottonseed oil
Aging Oxidants	Aging Oxidants	Aging Oxidants
Coffee Chocolate drinks\shakes Dark sodas Alcohol Tea (common black)	Deli meats Highly processed meats Highly spiced meats	Margarine Vegetable shortening Animal fats Cholesterol-free fatty foods

AGING HEALTHFULLY FOOD CHOICES

CARB's	FRUITS	VEGETABLES
1st Choice	**1st Choice**	**1st Choice**
Brown rice	Peach	Daikon
Wild rice	Pear	Burdock
Amaranth	Cherries	Red radish
Millet	Berries	Squash
Artichoke	Avocado	Chinese cabbage
Quinoa	Papaya	Turnips
Tapioca	Guava	Shiitake mushrooms
Milo	Persimmon	Lotus root
Tofu	Pomegranate	Ginger
Tempeh	Rhubarb	Green beans
Spelt	Prune	Carrot
Kamut	Apple	Collards
Teff	Figs	Kale
Sunflower seeds		Spinach
Sesame seeds		Artichoke
Pumpkin seeds		Asparagus
		Beets
		Brussels sprouts
		Broccoli, cauliflower
		Celery, cucumber
		Garlic, okra, peas
		Cabbage
2nd Choice	**2nd Choice**	**2nd Choice**
Rye	Lemon	Romaine lettuce
Buckwheat	Lime	Iceberg lettuce
Oats	Raisins	Boston lettuce
Potato	Watermelon	Onion
Barley	Kiwi	Red peppers
Yam	Grapefruit	Green peppers
	Cantaloupe	Eggplant
	Banana	Tomato
		Mushrooms
3rd Choice	**3rd Choice**	**3rd Choice**
Wheat	Orange	None
Corn	Pineapple	
White rice	Coconut	
Cashews	Strawberries	
Brazil nuts	Grapes	
Chestnuts	Honeydew	
Pecans	Mangoes	
Peanuts	Dates	
Walnuts	Polished fruits	
Almonds	Dried fruits	
Aging Oxidants	**Aging Oxidants**	**Aging Oxidants**
Sugar	None	None

ORGANIC VEGETABLE JUICES

Fresh organic vegetable juice is the very best way to assure an ample supply of nutrients for optimal function of enzymes of human energy, detoxification, digestive/absorptive, and neurotransmitter pathways. Such nutrients include:

1. Minerals 2. Vitamins 3. Enzymes.

For times when fresh juicing is not feasible, bottled organic vegetable juices may be used. Such juices contain all the minerals present in fresh juices (minerals do not degrade with storage). However, bottled juices may not contain many of the vitamins and enzymes present in fresh vegetables.

PEROXIDE-SALT BATH

(Please read this protocol twice before using it.)

First Bath

1. Fill the bathtub with warm water at a temperature you prefer.
2. Add one quart of 3% hydrogen peroxide to the bathtub.
3. Add one-half teaspoon of sea salt to the bath water (Baleine is a good brand.)
4. Avoid direct contact of the bathtub water with eyes.
5. After five minutes, add a second one-quart bottle of 3% hydrogen peroxide to the bath water, if no tissue irritation is experienced (see caution note below).
6. After five minutes, add the third quart bottle of 3% hydrogen peroxide to the bath water.
7. Stay in the bath from 20 to 25 minutes.

Second and Later Baths

1. Fill the bathtub with warm water at a temperature you prefer.
2. Add three one-quart bottles of 3% hydrogen peroxide to the bathtub.
3. Avoid direct contact of the bathtub water with eyes.
4. Stay in the bath from 20 to 25 minutes.

Caution:

1. Use bath water temperature that is comfortable for you.

2. Some women with symptoms of vaginitis may experience temporary irritation and may need to use only one-half or one bottle of peroxide until tissue irritation clears up.
3. Some persons experience lightheadedness if they stand up suddenly after a warm bath. It is a necessary safety step that this possibility be kept in mind and one should get up slowly, holding the safety bar or the side of the bathtub.

Note:

Brown-colored one quart bottles of 3% hydrogen peroxide are generally available from drug stores and other stores, such as A&P. It pays to do comparative shopping.

LIVER CASTOR OIL PACK AND LIVER FLUSH PROTOCOL

Two natural therapies that have stood the test of time for liver detoxification are liver castor oil pack and liver flush protocols. As for other specific therapies. I recommend that both liver pack and flush should be undertaken under professional supervision first. I myself prescribe castor oil liver packs to facilitate liver detox and reduce liver congestion as a part of our basic bowel-blood-liver detox program in most patients with chronic ailments.

Steps for the Castor Oil Liver Pack

1. Gently massage the *entire* liver area (upper abdomen and lower chest on the right side) along with the front of the lower abdomen with your left hand for two to four minutes.
2. Prepare a piece of flannel or cotton cloth large enough to cover the liver and abdomen areas when folded twice.
3. Fold flannel or cotton piece and soak it with castor oil (available from most pharmacies).
4. Cover the liver and abdominal areas with the soaked flannel or cotton piece and cover the cloth with a plastic sheet (an opened plastic bag is adequate). Use tape to anchor the plastic sheet.
5. Put a heating pad over as much of the area as possible covered by the pack, favoring the area of the liver. *The heating pad mustbe warm, not hot.*
6. Leave the castor oil soak for two hours, unless otherwise specified by your physician.
7. Gently wash off the castor oil with a mild soap after finishing the protocol.

Steps for One-Day Liver Flush

1. Drink 5 to 8 (or more if tolerated) glasses of organic apple cider or juice throughout the day. Persons with hypoglycemia or glucose intolerance may substitute organic vegetable juice for apple juice.
2. Drink additional water to maintain a state of overhydration from morning till 6 PM.
3. Take a vegetarian lunch at noon.
4 Continue with your prescribed nutrient and herbal supplements.
5. Three hours after lunch, take two teaspoons of disodium phosphate (or Epsom salt, if disodium phosphate is not available) dissolved in two ounces of hot water. Drink one cup of hot water with a few drops of lemon juice and a pinch of salt to eliminate bad taste from mouth.
6. Two hours later, repeat the above step (# 5).
7. Take an evening meal of grapefruit. (Grapefruit juice may be substituted if the whole fruit is not available. Fresh juice is preferred to canned juice.)
8. At bedtime, drink one cup of an equal-parts mixture of extra-virgin olive oil and lemon juice (1/2 cup of each). Again, fresh juice is preferred.
9. Lie in bed on your right side with knees pulled up for about 30 minutes.
10. Additional vegetarian meals may be taken if needed.
11. Be prepared to experience nausea, some abdominal cramps, and diarrhea during or after taking lemon juice and olive oil. You may need a Tigan suppository if nausea persists (prescription required from your physician).

Steps for Two-Day Liver Flush

1. Drink 5 to 8 (or more if tolerated) glasses of organic apple cider/juice or vegetable juice daily for two days.
2. Three hours after a vegetarian lunch on the second day, take 2 teaspoons of disodium phosphate dissolved in two ounces of hot water. Drink one cup of hot water with a few drops of lemon juice and a pinch of salt to eliminate bad taste from the mouth.
3. Continue with additional steps as for the one-day protocol (steps # 6 to 11).

MINI LIVER FLUSH PROTOCOL

One-half cup of fresh lemon juice
1 tsp olive oil
Dash of cayenne

BOWEL ECOLOGY PROTOCOLS

BOWEL ECOLOGY PROTOCOL #1®
One billion spores of *Lactobacillus acidophilus, Lactobacillus bulgaricus, bifidobacterium in a base of-complex vegetable fiber*, magnesium sulfate, vitamin b complex, L-histidine, L-arginine, pantethine, aloe vera.
BOWEL ECOLOGY PROTOCOL #2®
Alfalfa 500 mg, Pau d' arco 100 mg, Allium 100 mg, Licorice root extract 200 mg.
BOWEL ECOLOGY PROTOCOL #3®
Calcium 50 mg, Magnesium 50 mg, Grapefruit seed extract 25 mg, Aloe vera 1 mg, Spirulina 10 mg.
BOWEL ECOLOGY PROTOCOL #4®
Grapefruit seed extract 50 mg, Allium 50 mg, Pau d' a rco 500 mg.
BOWEL ECOLOGY PROTOCOL #5®
Par-quing 150 mg, Pau d' arco 150 mg, Beet root fiber 200 mg, Guar gum 100 mg.
BOWEL ECOLOGY PROTOCOL #6®
Echinacea 200 mg, Goldenseal root 150 mg, Astragalus root 150 mg, Burdock root 150 mg.
BOWEL ECOLOGY PROTOCOL #7®
Cascara sagrada 250 mg, Alfalfa 50 mg, Beet root fiber 50 mg, Goldenseal root 50 mg.
BOWEL ECOLOGY PROTOCOL #8®
Beet root fiber 700 mg.
BOWEL ECOLOGY PROTOCOL #9®
Milk thistle extract 200 mg, Goldenseal root 150 mg, Turmeric 150 mg, Jerusalem artichoke 150 mg.
BOWEL ECOLOGY PROTOCOL #10®
Vitamin B-5 165 mg, Folic acid 50 mcg, Pantethine 100 mg, PABA 5 mg, Potassium 2 mg, L-arginine HCI 25 mg, L-histidine 25 mg, L-ornithine 5 mg, Aloe vera 5 mg, Licorice Root 50 mg, Spirulina 10 mg.
BOWEL ECOLOGY PROTOCOL #11®
Senna 50 mg, Psyllium 400 mg, Beet root 100 mg, Glycerin 50 mg.
BOWEL ECOLOGY PROTOCOL #12®
Magnesium 150 mg, Potassium 50 mg, Taurine 250 mg.
BOWEL ECOLOGY PROTOCOL #13®
Fenugreek, Fennel seeds, Pau D'Arco, Licorice Powder
BOWEL ECOLOGY PROTOCOL #14®
Psyllium husk powder 4000 mg, Applepectin 100 mg

BLOOD ECOLOGY PROTOCOLS

BLOOD ECOLOGY PROTOCOL #1®
Cayenne 150 mg, Turmeric 150 mg, Garlic 150 mg, Dandelion root 150 mg, Ginger 150 mg.
BLOOD ECOLOGY PROTOCOL #2®
Butcher's broom 150 mg, Hawthorne 150 mg, Mother's wort 150 mg, St. John's wort 150 mg, Bilberry 150 mg.

BLOOD ECOLOGY PROTOCOL #3®
Siberian ginseng 150 mg, Mistletoe 150 mg, Linden flowers 150 mg, Schisandra 150 mg, Cranberry 150 mg.

LIVER ECOLOGY PROTOCOLS

LIVER ECOLOGY PROTOCOL #1®
Dandelion root 100 mg; Beet root fiber 50 mg; Black radish 50 mg; Goldenseal 50 mg; Catnip 50 mg; Methionine 400 mg; Choline bitartrate 200 mg; Inositol 20 mg.
LIVER ECOLOGY PROTOCOL #2®
Turmeric 100 mg; Milk thistle 100 mg; Red clover 100 mg; Ginger root 100 mg; Goldenseal 100 mg; Jerusalem artichoke 100 mg; Fennel seed 100 mg.

Abnormal Cellular Oxygen Metabolism in the September Canaries

The oxygen metabolism in the September canaries is abnormal. In simple words, cells suffer due to lack of functional oxygen. The enzymes involved in oxygen metabolism are impaired. Organic acids produced in the body are not broken down completely and accumulate in the cells. Dysfunctional oxygen metabolism is my term for such abnormalities of cellular oxygen metabolism. It is not merely a lack of oxygen, which is called anoxia in medical terminology. This is an important distinction.

The insight that dysfunctional oxygen metabolism was the fundamental molecular lesion in the September canaries came through my work with a very large number of air-hungry Gulf War, chronic fatigue, and fibromyalgia canaries. My studies with their blood and urine samples led me to conclude that their air hunger was neither imagined nor caused by a lack of oxygen due to disorders of the lung, heart, or blood (anemia). Rather, their basic problem was *dysfunctional* oxygen metabolism developing at a *cellular* level so that they could not properly *metabolize* oxygen, which they did breathe in. That was a major insight for me.

Anoxia is a lack of oxygen in tissues in conditions when oxygen metabolism itself is *normal*. For example, during an asthma attack, a person is short of breath and air-hungry because his bronchial tubes are in spasm and he cannot breathe in enough air. That condition creates anoxia. The *cellular* oxygen metabolism in asthma is normal, hence as soon as the bronchial spasm ends, the patient breathes easily and his air hunger disappears. The asthma sufferer looks completely normal within minutes of taking an inhaler treatment. There is no dysfunctional oxygen metabolism. That is not the case in fibromyalgia. If a fibro canary runs even seventy yards to catch a bus (assuming that he can do so), he may not be able to get out of his bed for a few days. That is so because oxygen metabolism in fibromyalgia is dysfunctional. As I indicated earlier, the September canaries commonly complained of air hunger or oxygen hunger. Many of them had consulted pulmonologists (lung specialists) for air hunger before they saw me. Their blood oxygen levels and other lung function test results were reported as "within normal limits." They were then told there was nothing wrong with them. Their pulmonologists had concluded that those canaries had only imagined their air hunger. In other words, they were malingerers—the old all-in-the-head theory. But, of course, the canaries were not imagining their air hunger. When they healed with proper treatment, the symptoms of air hunger or shortness of breath cleared up, indicating that the symptom of air hunger was a component of the total picture and was not merely imagined.

When proper laboratory tests are done, the September canaries showed clear evidence of abnormal oxygen metabolism. For example, tests for urinary organic acids show increased amounts of lactic acid and related compounds. That clearly indicates incomplete metabolism of sugars, proteins, and fats due to impaired oxygen metabolism. For professional and advanced readers, in Tables 1 to 2, I present data obtained in my study of eighty-four patients with oxygen dysfunction that demonstrate the various patterns and degrees of increased urinary excretion of organic acid. Following successful treatment of the underlying oxygen dysfunction, such patterns of abnormal organic acid excretion are normalized. Studies of blood samples with high-resolution microscopy also correlated well with both the clinical improvement and normalization of urine tests.

Table 1. The Frequency of Increased Urinary Excretion of Metabolites of the Krebs Cycle *Only* in 236 Patients with Dysfunctional Oxygen Metabolism	
Citric acid	196
Succinic acid	40
Aconitic acid	26
Fumaric acid	1
2-oxo-glutaric acid	0

Table 2. The Frequency of Increased Urinary Excretion of Metabolites of Gycolysis *Only* in 236 Patients with Dysfunctional Oxygen Metabolism	
Glyceric acid	59
2-hydroxybutyric acid	26
Lactic acid	12
Pyruvic acid	1

Impaired Immune Status in the September Canaries

The laboratory evidence for impaired immune status of the September canaries can be expediently established by a variety of tests. In general, two good approaches are the following:

1. Demonstration of suboptimal levels of protective antibodies; and
2. Detection of abnormal and harmful antibodies.

In the following two tables, I contrast a vigorous immune response to immunotherapy in a healthy child with a weakened immune response to similar therapy in a September canary. In Table 1, note the sharp rises in the quantities of protective antibodies following treatment, indicating a strong immune response. By contrast, the values for similar antibodies in a September canary show actual drops after the events of September Eleven, indicating immune injury.

Table 1. Robust Immune Response to Immunotherapy in a Healthy Child (Compare with Table 2)		
Allergen	**Pre-Treatment**	**Posttreatment**
Date	11/18/92	08/09/93
BERMUDA GRASS	83	783
JUNE GRASS	128	708
SHORT RAGWEED	186	1,093
PLANTAIN	1,454	1,958
BOX ELDER (MAPLE)	660	1,194
SYCAMORE	324	403
ALTERNARIA	2,041	2,046
PENICILLIUM	2,362	2,542
CANDIDA	2,554	2,596
CAT EPITHELIUM	1,098	1,524

Other works by Majid Ali, M.D.:

The Cortical Monkey and Healing, 1991

The Butterfly and Life Span Nutrition, 1992

The Ghorra and Limbic Exercise, 1993

The Canary and Chronic Fatigue, 1994

RDA: Rats, Drugs and Assumptions, 1995

What Do Lions Know About Stress, 1996

Healing, Miracles and the Bite of the Grey Dog, 1998

Oxygen and Aging, 2000

The Canary and Fibromyalgia, 2003